THE 28-DAY
KETO
CURE

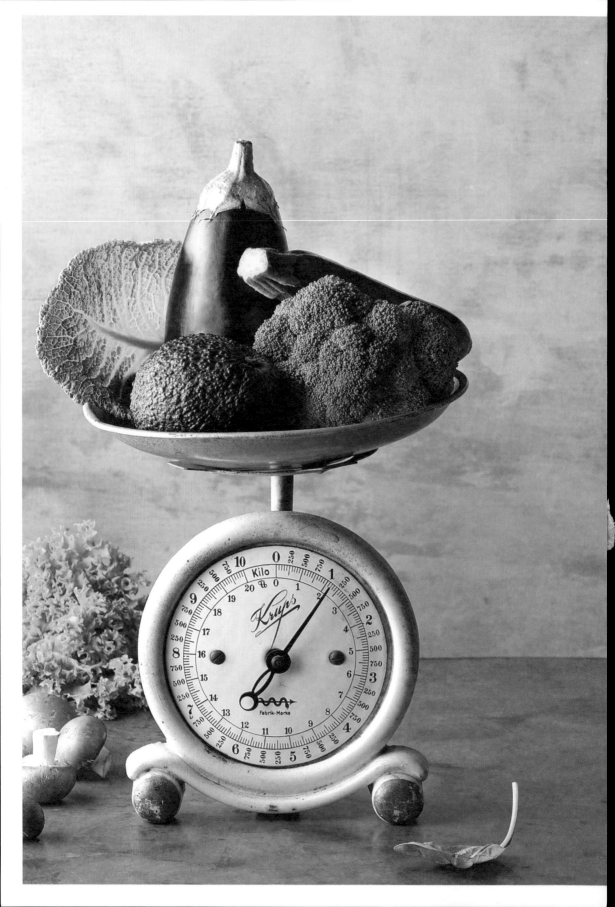

THE 28-DAY KETO CURE

The Essential LOW-CARB, HIGH-FAT, WEIGHT LOSS PLAN for a Healthier Life

JÜRGEN VORMANN, PhD
with NICO STANITZOK

STERLING EPICURE
New York

CONTENTS

The (v) beside a recipe title identifies a vegetarian dish

FOREWORD

I first studied nutritional science over 30 years ago and have been researching and teaching it ever since. In hardly any other field of science has our understanding of what is healthy for us changed as fundamentally as in relation to nutrition.

For a long time, a low-fat diet was considered synonymous with being healthy. People cut back on fat and made up for lost calories by eating (supposedly healthier) carbohydrates. Then, research started to show that a high-carb diet has the potential to lead to serious health complications, such as obesity and type 2 diabetes, two of the most prevalent health problems in modern society. As a result, the low-carbohydrate diet became a highly popular alternative.

But eating fat to stay slim? Well, yes. Today we know that a high-fat diet can actually be beneficial, particularly if you are overweight. While it understandably feels counterintuitive to eat more fat, the latest scientific evidence shows that a low-carbohydrate high-fat diet combined with exercise will help regulate your metabolism and give you back control over your weight.

Because eating habits are shaped and consolidated over long periods of time, it can be difficult for us to make the fundamental shift from a carbohydrate-based to a high-fat diet—not least because of a lack of kitchen inspiration. This is where we come in. In *The 28-Day Keto Cure* we will help you adapt to the Low-Carb High-Fat diet (LCHF for short), with plenty of delicious recipes to show you the way. My friend and colleague Nico Stanitzok has based his career on his passion for tasty, nutritionally-balanced food. For this book he has developed recipes suitable for everyday life which are low in carbs, high in fat, and will keep you satisfied and healthy.

This book, and our 28-day program, is a starting point. People who want to lose weight will see the results quickly but the main benefit for everyone is that this is a medium- to long-term healthy diet-option, in contrast to the low-carb, high-protein diet which has several negative impacts on general health. In the pages that follow, you will discover why the LCHF approach is the key to successful weight loss.

Professor Jürgen Vormann

WHY LOW CARB HIGH FAT?

In order for our bodies to function properly, our diet has to include a regular supply of energy from one of three sources: carbohydrate, fat, and protein. If we restrict one of the nutrients in this mix, but want to maintain the same energy intake, we have to make up the shortfall by consuming more of one of the other energy sources.

Some low-carb diets rely on substituting protein for the missing carbohydrate calories—so you might eat some extra steak in place of pasta or bread. The abundance of meat has made this diet attractive to many people, especially men, at least for a time. But there are certain pitfalls that can limit the benefits of these kinds of diets; when the amino acids that make up the proteins are broken down, the body produces intermediate products that form carbohydrates. The end result of this is that consuming too much protein indirectly increases your supply of carbohydrates. High protein consumption can also put a strain on the body's acid-base balance.

MORE FAT, LESS PROTEIN

If we don't substitute the calories missing from carbohydrates with protein, the only other option is fat. In a low-carb diet, your body burns more of its own fat stores, which is exactly the effect you want if you are trying to lose weight. Reducing your carbohydrate intake means your muscle cells in particular burn more fat to generate energy. The heart, for instance, can derive almost all its energy requirements from fatty acids.

A low-carb high-fat (LCHF) diet has an additional advantage over the low-carb high-protein diet: by increasing the intake of fat at the same time as limiting carbohydrates, it pushes the body to produce ketones. In a traditional diet, these chemicals are only present in the body in tiny quantities. But they are an effective substitute for carbohydrates, and all cells can use ketones as a rapid form of fuel.

Since we usually have substantial fat stores in our bodies, it is always possible for our body to produce ketones. However, ketones are only created when the body's metabolism switches to fat burning, particularly in the liver. As soon as we start consuming significant quantities of carbohydrates, our metabolism switches back to using glucose; once this occurs, we start building up fat stores again and ketosis ceases. Reducing your carbohydrate consumption in the short term will not produce a long-term effect, so the crucial thing for maintaining your target weight is to reduce carbohydrates on a sustained basis.

Decades of warnings against excessive fat consumption have certainly made their mark. Many of us who want to lose weight find it counterintuitive to increase our fat intake. But this diet has already helped a great many people; it will help you, too.

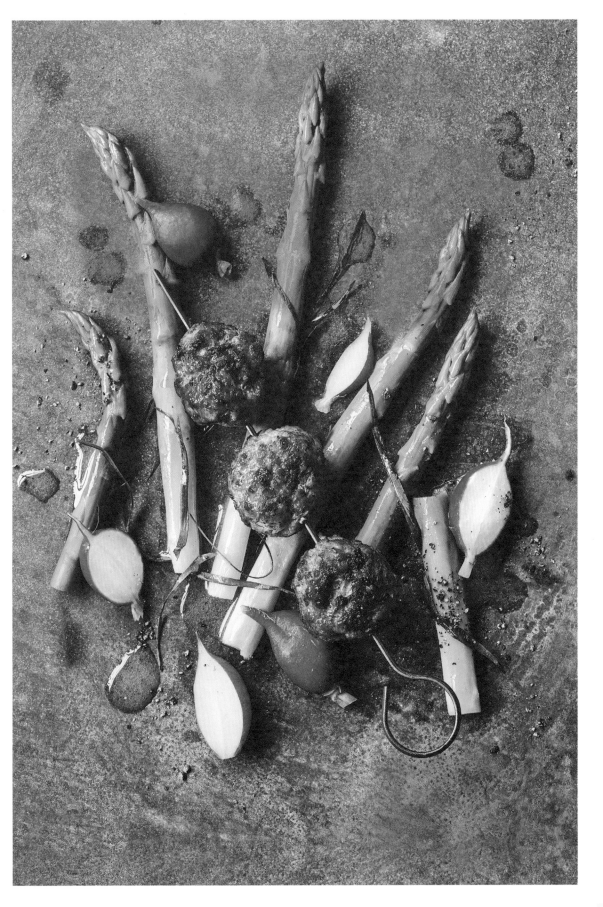

FATTENING CARBOHYDRATES

Carbohydrates are absolutely essential for our metabolism. But in excess quantities they overwhelm our blood sugar levels and encourage our bodies to store fat. In order to lose weight, we have to address carbohydrate consumption.

Our metabolism releases insulin to control blood sugar concentrations, ensuring there is always enough glucose in our bloodstream while also preventing excess. Any excess sugar in the blood is rapidly removed—our muscles then burn (and store some of) this glucose. But if we continue to supply the body with glucose, for example, in the case of a carbohydrate-rich meal, then we hit the scenario we want to avoid: the excess sugar is no longer stored as carbohydrates and is instead converted into fat.

Often the food we eat does not consist purely of carbohydrates; it also contains fat. In this case, our metabolism has enough glucose available that it does not need to use the fat we are eating as a source of energy—so off it goes, straight into our fat stores. Only once glucose levels in our bloodstream are back to normal can our body use this fat. However, a decrease in blood sugar will send an unmistakable signal to our body that additional supplies are required: we become hungry. If we then eat more carbohydrates, our body uses these first and the stored fat stays in our fatty tissues. It's a vicious circle that ultimately leads to obesity. Of course, you can break the cycle by refusing to give in to your hunger—but this is far from easy. Or you can stimulate glucose consumption through exercise, but in order to lose weight successfully, physical activity needs to supplement an existing calorie deficit.

INSULIN AS THE CONTROLLER

The hormone insulin plays a central role in controlling glucose metabolism. It enables glucose to be absorbed by the cells in our muscles and liver and ensures that the metabolic processing in our brain functions correctly. Whenever glucose enters our bloodstream following a meal, the pancreas releases insulin to channel that glucose into our cells and inhibit fat burning. After a carbohydrate-rich meal, our body produces a lot of insulin, which continues to act in the bloodstream even after many hours. This means that if we want to program our metabolism to burn fat, it is crucial to keep insulin levels as low as possible. This also helps protect our capacity to produce insulin. If we push our body to produce a lot of insulin over a sustained period, the result can be insulin resistance, where the metabolism barely responds, or fails to respond at all, to insulin. This leads to obesity and diabetes.

LESS IS MORE

Simply put, the fewer carbs you eat, the better! On the LCHF diet, only about 1¾ ounces (50 grams) of carbohydrates per day are needed to meet the brain's requirements. When resting, our brain requires roughly 20 percent of the calories we consume—for 2000 calories per day, that amounts to about 400 calories. This corresponds to approximately 3½ ounces (100 grams) of carbohydrates. As we reprogram our metabolic system, the absolute glucose requirement (the minimum amount needed for brain function) falls to roughly 1¾ ounces (50 grams) because around half of the brain's energy needs can be met indirectly by breaking down fat. Individuals vary in terms of their metabolism and energy requirements, but over time you will find out what your minimum requirements are.

NOT ALL CARBS ARE BAD

It's not just a question of how many carbohydrates foods contain, but also how quickly each particular carbohydrate is converted into glucose in the bloodstream. This is called a food's glycemic index, which describes how quickly the carbohydrates in any food are broken down in the intestine and channeled into the blood.

The guidelines are relatively simple: Cereal products, potatoes, rice, and sugar are prohibited or only to be consumed in very small quantities. Carbohydrates should really come almost exclusively from vegetables, salad, and a bit of fruit—these are the "good" carb sources (see page 12).

HIDDEN CARBOHYDRATES

Ready-made sauces, yogurts, and juices often contain carbohydrates where you would least expect them. They are also found in sausages, shop-bought meatballs, fish dishes, and in any products coated in breadcrumbs. Even pulses and sweet fruit contain considerable quantities. If you eat carbohydrates these should ideally come from vegetables and fruit, rather than from grains and potatoes. But you should also be wary of hidden carbs. Oysters for example—unlike other fish—have a relatively high carb count at five percent. So do garlic and onions. Always check the labeling on processed foods: you may be surprised to see where the carbs are coming from.

Be careful with prepared foods such as egg salad, dressings and sauces: Sugar is often added as a flavour enhancer. The more processed the product, the greater the likelihood it will contain hidden carbohydrates in the form of sugar and starch. A salad, often considered a healthy alternative, may actually become a calorie and carbohydrate trap because of its dressing. To be on the safe side, prepare sauces and dressings yourself, and check the ingredients when you eat out in restaurants. Ketchup is a whopping 25 percent carbs. While fruit is an important component of the LCHF diet, bear in mind that not all fruits are equal. Pears, for example, are 12 percent carb. While bananas—that sports person's favorite—are actually 20 percent carb.

Nuts make a quick and easy snack for in-between meals, and on-the-go. Since nuts are naturally very high in calories, it is important to pay attention to the quantities. Macadamia nuts are ideal for a ketogenic diet, being particularly high in fat whilst comparatively low in carbohydrate, making them a great source of energy. Brazil nuts and almonds are also good options, but some nuts, such as walnuts, should be consumed in moderation and others, like cashews, avoided completely.

GOOD CARBOHYDRATES

If you are going to consume carbohydrates, wherever possible these should come from vegetables and fruit. Here you'll find the carbohydrate sources that fit best in a LCHF diet.

① FRUIT

Contains important vitamins and minerals that are essential on a LCHF diet. They also provide us with other healthy substances such as antioxidants. This is particularly the case for strongly colored varieties of fruit, like berries, papaya, or apricots. Simple reminder: The sweeter the fruit, the less suitable it is for LCHF. Older apple or pear varieties, which can be found at farmer's markets for instance, usually contain less sugar than newer varieties that have been cultivated for their high sugar content. Quinces are also relatively low in sugar. The same is true of citrus fruits such as grapefruits and lemons. Make sure you eat fruit that has been processed as little as possible, because all too often sugar is added during processing. Frozen fruit is great, too, as it is harvested when perfectly ripe. Frozen berries are a particularly wonderful daily addition to the menu and have a high nutritional value.

② VEGETABLES

Contain lots of vitamins, minerals, and alkaline substances that are particularly important on a LCHF diet. The daily quantity of carbohydrates should be derived predominantly from vegetables. All types of cabbage, green salad, cucumbers, spinach, tomatoes, asparagus, broccoli, eggplant, zucchini, bell peppers, onions, and mushrooms can be eaten freely. Take advantage of the high fat content of avocados and olives. Frozen vegetables are a healthy and practical alternative to fresh produce. Be more restrained when it comes to root vegetables, such as potatoes, yams, beets, and carrots, because plants store carbohydrates in roots and bulbs.

③ PULSES

Are a good source of high-quality protein, but lentils and chickpeas in particular also contain lots of carbohydrates. If pulses are to be on the menu, you should preferably stick to peas and beans, which are lower in carbohydrates than other pulses.

④ ALTERNATIVE FLOURS

Can replace carbohydrate-rich ingredients such as sugar, potatoes, rice, and cereals, which are less suitable for the LCHF diet. Almond flour is a great flour substitute that contains just 6 grams (about ¼ ounce) of carbohydrates per 2½ ounces (100g). You can use it with sweeteners in baked items, though you will find that your appetite for sweet things gradually diminishes over time. Other nut flours such as ground linseed, pumpkin seeds, or pine nuts are also good alternatives to cereal flours.

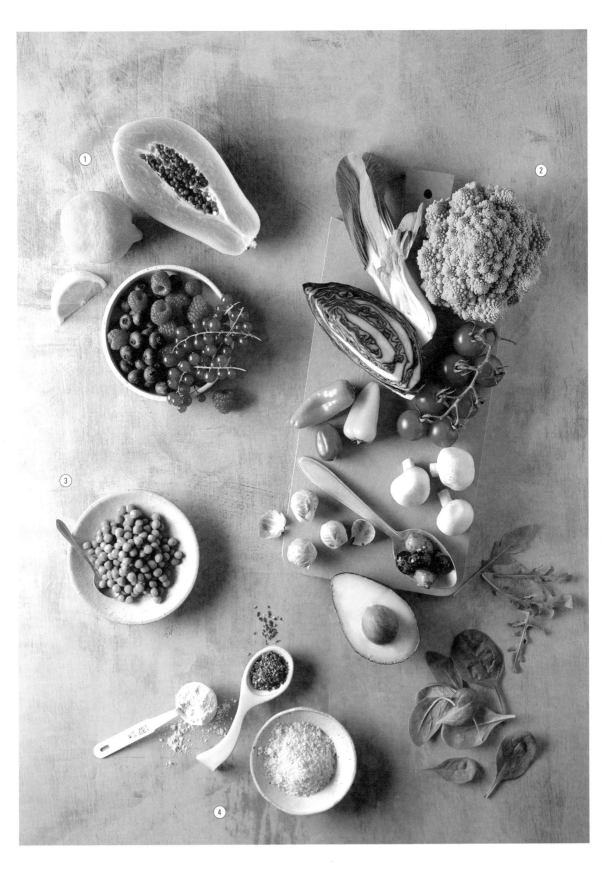

EAT PROTEIN SPARINGLY

It's tempting to make up for the calories saved on carbohydrates in the form of large portions of meat, fish, or cheese. But this results in a far higher protein consumption than the roughly 1 gram per kilo (about 2¼ ounces) of body weight required each day. On a low-carb diet, the upper limit should be around 2 grams protein per kilo body weight. And this can be reached in no time: For someone weighing 165 pounds (75 kilos), this works out at roughly 5 ounces (150 grams) protein. When expressed in calories, this corresponds to roughly 600 per day.

THE DARK SIDE OF PROTEINS

Proteins are composed of individual components known as amino acids. We need amino acids as fuel and as a building material, for example for our muscles. Amino acids contain certain chemical elements, especially nitrogen and sulfur, which have to be excreted via the kidneys because we cannot convert everything into endogenous protein (protein that ensures cells function correctly). This is why excess protein intake puts a strain on our kidneys. A diet based exclusively on protein is actually impossible in the long term, as our kidneys have a limited ability to eliminate nitrogen.

The sulfur contained in protein poses additional problems. Sulfur can only be eliminated from the body in the form of sulfuric acid via the kidneys. Excess quantities of sulfuric acid can contribute significantly to harmful hyperacidity in the body. From around age 30 the excretion capacity of our kidneys becomes more limited, and from this point on there is an unavoidable reduction in kidney capacity of approximately 1 percent for each year of life.

Due to this continual decline in kidney function, older people can be particularly affected by excess acidity and its negative consequences. The body attempts to compensate for any hyperacidity by releasing more and more alkaline components from the bone structure. Unfortunately, this also results in vital calcium being lost from the bones; the risk of osteoporosis increases and the bones become less stable. An exposure to acidity can also result in painful changes to connective tissue. Ketones are also acidic, which means the aim must be to keep the quantity of additional acid produced to a minimum.

For this reason, a LCHF diet with high quantities of protein is ill-advised. There is another important reason, too: Some of the amino acids that make up proteins can be converted into glucose. The proportion of these amino acids is the same across all foods containing protein, so it isn't possible to specifically avoid these proteins. Just like carbohydrates, they can also trigger an insulin response—an effect we want to avoid.

High protein intake is often synonymous with high levels of meat consumption. In addition to animal protein, this means that large quantities of nucleic acids are consumed, and when these are broken down uric acid is produced. This can lead to problems when converting to a LCHF diet, because ketones and uric acid end up competing for the same excretion systems in the kidneys. This can result in obstructions and inhibit excretion. So, at the start of a LCHF diet, the concentration of uric acid in the blood may increase. If a lot of meat is also consumed, the effect is further exacerbated.

Although uric acid is an important antioxidant in the blood and an increase is generally beneficial, this is not the case if you are already suffering from gout, as gout is caused by elevated uric acid levels. If this applies to you, please consult your physician before making any dietary changes. With normal protein intake, kidney function will adapt after four to six weeks and uric acid levels will normalize.

Increased protein intake is possible on a low-carb regime, but not to the extent that would be required to make up for the calorie deficit caused by omitting carbohydrates. Only higher fat consumption can do this.

SLIMMING WITH FAT?

It seems obvious why the original aim for losing weight was to eat less fat. After all, 1 gram of fat contains more than double the calories of either carbohydrates or protein. By reducing fat, you can cut back on significantly more calories than through the same quantity of proteins or carbohydrates. However, we now know that fat is particularly crucial for feeling full. The same quantity of calories in the form of carbohydrates is significantly less filling than those from fat.

Fat has long been blamed for causing various health conditions, especially heart disease. However, we have now established that important research in this area was misinterpreted. For many decades, people have been attempting to lower high cholesterol values (regarded as the main cause of heart attacks) by reducing fat intake. Blood cholesterol levels can be reduced in this way, but this also impacts HDL cholesterol, which we now regard as beneficial to our health. Based on current knowledge, a diet that is high in fat and low in carbohydrates does not constitute a risk in terms of cardiovascular disease. Whether it actually reduces the general risk is a question requiring further research—but initial scientific studies certainly point in this direction.

NOT ALL FATS ARE EQUAL

Needless to say, the kind of fat you eat is hugely important: not all fats are equal. The very fats that have so long been stigmatized are ideally suited for the LCHF diet thanks to their special metabolic state. Long, medium, or short-chain? Saturated or unsaturated? These terms crop up repeatedly in association with fats. But what do they mean?

In terms of their chemical make-up, fatty acids are described with reference to the length of their chains, on the one hand, and the nature of their bonds, on the other. Fats with single bonds are described as saturated, while those with double bonds are categorized as unsaturated fats. Chain length and bonding characteristics don't just determine the chemical characteristics of fats, they are also relevant when it comes to nutritional value. One indicator of what kind of fat we are dealing with is its consistency: Fats with a higher proportion of unsaturated, long-chain fatty acids are liquid at room temperature, those with saturated fatty acids are solid.

UNSATURATED FATTY ACIDS

Unsaturated fatty acids are important for our metabolism and are known to be beneficial for our health. These include the omega-3 group of fatty acids, but also the monounsaturated oleic acids (of which there are particularly large quantities in olive oil) and the doubly unsaturated linoleic acids (especially prevalent in safflower and grape-seed oil). Omega-3 fatty acids have a particularly beneficial impact on cell membrane structure: these are found in oily sea fish.

Another important source of omega-3 fatty acids is offered by milk, dairy products, meat, sausage, bacon and other products from animals that are allowed to graze on natural pasture. Omega-3 fatty acids from grass are concentrated in these foods, which is why butter from pasture-reared cows also contains a significant proportion of these healthy fats. In addition, olive oil is good for us because of its high levels of monounsaturated oleic acids.

Maintaining a good balance in our diet between plenty of omega-3 fatty acids and minimal omega-6 fatty acids keeps us healthy and protects against illnesses such as cardiovascular disease and arteriosclerosis. Even once conditions like this have developed, and their associated symptoms of inflammation and pain are evident (as with rheumatism, for instance), a high intake of omega-3 with restricted omega-6 fatty acids can have a beneficial impact. Sufficient quantities of omega-3 fatty acids can significantly inhibit the formation of certain pain mediators, known as prostaglandins.

SATURATED FATTY ACIDS

A certain notoriety has been acquired by fats with saturated fatty acids, which are chemically stable and barely change when heated. These fats are claimed to have a negative impact on cholesterol levels, but with LCHF these effects are avoided as the fats are broken down very quickly to produce energy.

As a result, animal products with saturated fats from butter, lard, or bacon can be safely included in a LCHF diet. Saturated fats are rare in the plant domain. There are only two varieties with a high proportion of unsaturated fats that are relevant from a nutritional perspective: coconut oil and palm kernel oil (not to be confused with palm oil).

MCT FATS

Medium-chain fatty acids, or MCTs for short, offer a crucial benefit for the LCHF diet: They have an exceptional capacity to be absorbed very quickly from the stomach and converted into ketones in the liver. These fats enable the desired ketosis to be achieved significantly faster than with other fats.

Virgin coconut oil (preferably organic) is unrivaled in terms of its proportion of MCTs, with approximately 50 percent MCT fats. When it comes to the other fats we normally use, only butter has any significant quantity of medium-chain fatty acids (approx. 10 percent). Unfortunately, coconut oil is often classified as being unhealthy since it contains predominantly saturated fatty acids. In fact, we now know that not only is coconut fat metabolized very quickly and has a ketogenic effect, it also brings a variety of other health benefits.

OMEGA-6 FATTY ACIDS

Less favorable fats are those with a relatively high proportion of omega-6 fatty acids in comparison to omega-3 fatty acids. You should steer clear of popular oils such as safflower, wheat germ, rapeseed, soy, and sunflower, not to mention any margarines produced from these oils. Unhealthy artificial trans fats can be produced from these sources, especially if they are heated: This happens during food production when hydrogen is added to liquid vegetable oils in order to make them more solid. While you should aim to include some naturally-occurring trans fats in your diet—these are the fats found in grass-fed meats and dairy—the artificial variety is damaging to health, associated with an increased risk of heart disease and cholesterol.

GOOD FATS

Omega-3 fatty acids and MCTs offer a range of benefits for the LCHF diet. You should prioritize these when selecting which fats to eat. Make organic your first choice as the healthiest option.

① FROM GRAZING ANIMALS

For all animal products, from meat to milk, the proportion of omega-3 fatty acids is highly dependent on the animal fodder: Good fatty acids from fresh grass become concentrated in meat and milk. That is why it's important to focus on pasture-grazing or grass-fed animals. Lard is ideal for frying, and bacon contributes an irresistible, rounded flavor while also being rich in healthy fatty acids. Butter and cream are the only animal fats containing medium-chain fatty acids that can be swiftly converted into ketones. Both have a mellow taste and are really versatile: ideal natural flavor enhancers.

② FROM MARINE ANIMALS

High-fat sea fish, such as eel, mackerel, sardine, salmon, and herring are especially rich in omega-3 fatty acids. Once again, the proportion of these nutritious fatty acids depends on the food the animals eat. Targeted, species-appropriate feeding can be used to produce very high levels of healthy fatty acids. By contrast, farmed fish that are not fed with the species' requirements in mind are relatively low in in these substances. When buying fish and shellfish caught in the wild, make sure they have been fished sustainably, as indicated by the MSC seal of approval.

③ FROM PLANT SOURCES

Two features distinguish a good vegetable oil: the ratio of omega-3 to omega-6 fatty acids and the proportion of MCTs. In cold-pressed oils all the beneficial constituents, such as vitamins, are retained. Organically produced (virgin) coconut oil should be your first choice alongside lard for frying and baking. Olive oil is primarily used for cold dishes or as a flavoring agent drizzled over food. With its high proportion of oleic acids, it regulates the fat metabolism and reduces the level of toxic fats.

The same is true for avocado oil: It consists of 50 percent oleic acids. This oil adds a nutty element to vegetable and mushroom recipes, salads, and soups. Nut oils made from walnuts, hazelnuts, and macadamias are likewise suitable for cold dishes but not for cooking. These oils contain a well-balanced combination of healthy fats. Just a few drops are all that's needed to enhance salads, soups, and vegetable dishes. The distinctive flavor of linseed oil also goes beautifully with these dishes, though it must not be heated. With a 6:1 ratio of omega-3 to omega-6 fatty acids,it is pretty much ideal for the human metabolism.

KETONES AND KETOSIS

Fat consists of a glycerol structure to which three fatty acids are coupled. When fat is broken down, these acids are released and used by our muscular system to produce energy. What is left is the glycerol component from which glucose is formed.

If fat intake is high, the body cannot utilize all the fatty acids immediately. That's why it transports any excess into the liver to be converted into so-called ketones. Ketones are acids with one particularly pertinent characteristic: They can be quickly absorbed by all cells—even in nervous tissue and in the brain. This isn't the case for fats and fatty acids because they cannot penetrate the blood-brain barrier in the form in which they are transported.

The really special thing about keto acids is that our nerve cells can use them very easily as a source of energy, which reduces the need for glucose. If sufficient ketones are available, up to 60 percent of the brain's energy requirements can be met from this source. This also produces fewer free radicals as a potentially damaging by-product than when breaking down glucose (see page 10).

A high quantity of fat in our diet helps support brain function. Just a few weeks on a LCHF diet is almost always enough for there to be an adequate energy supply to our cells (at least for people with preexisting fat deposits). Since our hunger mechanism is constantly geared towards averting any potential energy deficit, this avoids triggering our innate alarm system and hunger is easily avoided.

DOWN WITH CARBOHYDRATES

In order to bring about these positive effects, it is essential to radically reduce your carbohydrate intake at the same time as you increase your fat intake. Only then can the right ketone concentration in the blood be achieved. On a diet with a high proportion of carbohydrates, there are practically no ketones in the blood and the brain uses glucose exclusively. Only once ketone levels rise above a value of 18 mg/dL (1 mmol/L) in the blood will ketones be used as described. This level will only be attained if carbohydrate consumption is significantly less than 3½ ounces (100 grams) per day, ideally only 1¾ ounces (50 grams).

The key to success with the LCHF diet is achieving ketosis. In this metabolic state, fat reserves are broken down without causing any hunger pangs. In this way, the brain continues to be supplied with energy even as glucose levels fall.

WHAT HAPPENS DURING KETOSIS?

Any glucose shortfall, and hence any energy deficit in the brain, inevitably leads to an intense feeling of hunger. Normally we give in to these hunger pangs and the energy deficit required to lose weight is never achieved.

But if we are able to put our bodies into ketosis, the brain never experiences this potential energy crisis and we simply don't feel hungry. Most people can then happily get by with just two meals a day. One positive side effect of this is that burning ketones results in fewer oxygen-free radicals, which can be particularly damaging to cell membranes. What's more, ketones actually strengthen the mechanisms to protect against oxidative stress and have a detoxifying impact on oxygen-free radicals.

KETONE CONCENTRATION

A good concentration of ketones in the blood should range from 18 to 54 mg/dL (1 to 3 mmol/L, see diagram on page 23). While it is possible to measure ketones in your blood, it is easier to use a urine test, which you can carry out using ketone test strips that can be found in drugstores. When first converting to the LCHF diet, this lets you check whether your reduction in carbohydrates has been sufficient to achieve ketosis.

MEASURING KETOSIS

When you start out on the LCHF diet, measure the ketone levels in your urine each morning. The easiest and least expensive way to do this is to use a testing strip. There are many brands available in health stores or online. Whichever you buy, read the product insert in detail but usually these are the best steps to follow:

Collect urine in a clean, dry container and dip the test strip in as far as possible. Wait for 15 seconds or whatever time is stated on the brand of test strips you are using. Compare the color on your strip to the color array on the side of the bottle.

Any color other than the original beige means there are some ketones in your urine. After a few days you should notice an increase in ketone concentrations in the urine. The closer the color is toward deep purple, the more ketones there are in your body. Generally a consistent low-mid level of ketosis is the best for weight loss and feeling good.

Incorporating coconut oil, in particular, will ensure that your ketone levels rise. If this is not evident after about a week, you will need to examine your diet again for concealed carbohydrates or a high-protein intake. In which case, you may need to restrict your carbohydrate consumption further in order to reprogram your metabolism.

At the end of the 28-day plan, you should notice that the ketone concentration in your urine has reduced. This does not mean that the LCHF diet is no longer working. Quite the opposite: it indicates that your metabolism has adapted to breaking down ketones and these are now predominantly being burned and no longer excreted.

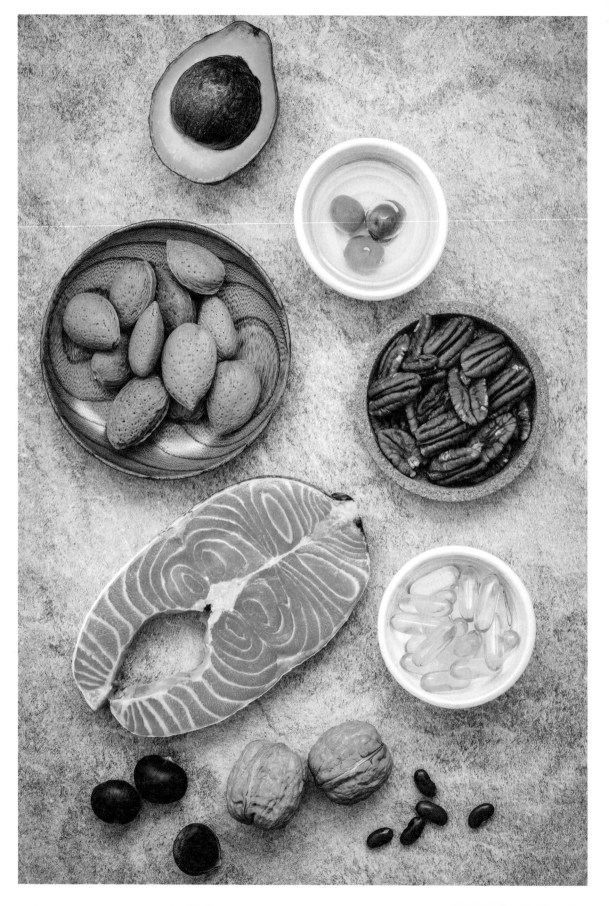

Optimal ketone concentrations should be between 18 and 54 mg/dL (1 and 3 mmol/L).

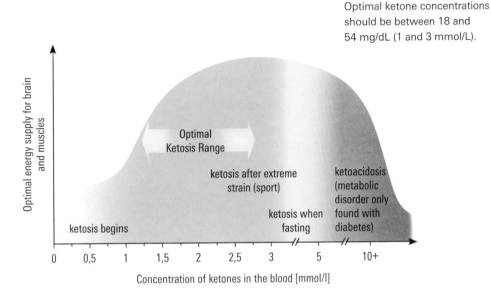

Concentration of ketones in the blood [mmol/l]

KETOSIS AND PERFORMANCE

If you can sustain ketosis in the long term, your athletic performance will also improve. Ketones provide muscles with a reliable energy supply, which means you can avoid the dreaded energy slump. This abrupt energy deficiency arises if there is a sharp drop in glucose concentration in the blood and insufficient ketones to compensate for the deficit. Ketosis also ensures a steady supply of energy to the brain, enhancing its function and making ketosis hugely significant for those suffering from dementia. Once the brain's carbohydrate metabolism can no longer operate adequately through insulin, ketones can provide the necessary energy instead.

It was established recently that Alzheimer's disease is also influenced by the same mechanism. Since insulin in the brains of those affected is no longer effective, scientists sometimes describe this form of dementia as "type 3 diabetes". As we know, ketones provide the brain with an alternative energy source and improve nerve function, and initial scientific research indicates significant improvements for dementia patients on a ketogenic diet.

DON'T GET YOUR TERMS CONFUSED

Ketosis is frequently confused with ketoacidosis, a life-threatening metabolic disorder found in diabetics. Ketone concentrations found in the blood of patients with this condition are ten times greater than those found in ketosis, but there is no way these kinds of ketone concentrations will be achieved purely through the LCHF diet.

1

THE 28-DAY PLAN

Welcome to the 28–day diet plan! You are going to enjoy delicious recipes every day and, as your body adapts to the new diet, you won't feel hungry or lethargic. As with any new diet, the best time to start is on a weekend so you can give yourself plenty of time to get organized. Remember to be kind to yourself and ask for support and understanding from those around you.

LOSING WEIGHT WITH THE LCHF PLAN

To lose weight with the LCHF diet, you will need to pay attention to your total calorie intake. Weigh yourself regularly for several weeks before you start the diet to check on your usual daily calorie requirement: If your weight remains constant, then your calorie intake corresponds roughly to your requirements. Check with your physician if you are unsure.

Calculating your BMI

Your Body Mass Index (BMI) is a good way to check your body fat ratio. To measure your own BMI, multiply your height in inches by itself. Then multiply your weight in pounds by 703. Divide your weight by your height. An ideal ratio is around 20-25 – over 30 is considered obese. More information can be found at:
www.nhlbi.nih.gov/health/educational/lose_wt/BMI/bmicalc.htm.

Your daily calorie requirement varies from person to person depending on your initial weight and how physically active you are. However, as a general rule, we can assume that for people with a body mass index of up to 30, reducing the daily calorie intake to approximately 1,500 calories for women and 2,000 calories for men will bring about steady weight loss. For someone with a significantly higher BMI, a higher calorie diet can still result in weight loss. On the 28-day plan, you want to ensure that your calorie intake is consistently lower than your daily calorie requirement.

With three recipes from the daily menu plan in this section you will consume roughly 1,500 calories per portion. This calorie intake can be increased, for example with smoothies or snacks, but take care to avoid the proportion of carbohydrates getting too high. Note that this book includes more great-tasting dishes than are included in the 28-day plan, giving you the inspiration to continue the LCHF diet and transform your lifestyle.

Twenty-eight days is a long time so you may not be eating all your meals at home. In restaurants, simply avoid the standard "filling sides" such as pasta, potatoes, rice, and bread. The ideal choice is some baked fish or a steak with a large salad—steer clear of the usual dressings and ask for some oil and vinegar or lemon juice. And of course, hearty portions of vegetables—preferably cooked in plenty of butter—are the perfect side dish.

SUPPLEMENTS AND ADDITIONS FOR THE 28-DAY PLAN

Top up your mineral stores

Once ketosis has been achieved, there is initially an increased excretion of minerals together with water. The best way to compensate for any potential mineral deficiencies is with meat or vegetable stock. Eat plenty of vegetables to get adequate magnesium, which is required for almost all of our body's biochemical functions. Increase your magnesium intake to start with, preferably with citrate-based supplements.

Where there is acidity....

...you need alkalinity. To keep pH values in the bloodstream constant, ketones (which are acids in terms of their chemistry) must be balanced out with appropriate alkaline substances. Vegetables and vegetable stock are good alkaline sources. If protein intake is increased at the same time, acidity levels in the blood will increase even further and consumption of alkaline foodstuffs alone will often not be sufficient to compensate. The best thing is to take alkaline, citrate-based mineral supplements (see page 30).

Bulletproof breakfast power

The perfect drink for those who refuse to eat breakfast or who are grouchy in the morning is bulletproof coffee. This is coffee enriched with butter and/or coconut oil and will fuel you with energy until midday. Not only does it fill you up, it also catapults you into the day feeling super fit. To keep things varied, why not try some cocoa with warming spices instead of coffee or tweak your coffee to suit your personal taste (see recipes on pages 170 and 171)?

Alcohol?

The good news is that alcoholic drinks are not banned. But beer is best avoided—not for nothing is it sometimes referred to as liquid bread! A glass of dry white wine is certainly permitted, likewise spirits as long as you steer clear of sweet liqueurs. Try some vodka or gin mixed with a large glass of mineral water and a dash of lime juice.

THE DAY BEFORE YOU START

The day before you start, go shopping and get everything ready in the kitchen. Clean out your refrigerator and store cupboard of anything you won't need. Don't buy any fast food or packaged food and prepare your first breakfast the evening before if you can, so you can take the time to enjoy it. If you are a vegetarian, or simply want to go vegetarian while on the LCHF 28-day diet plan, then substitute the meat-based recipes in the planner with any of the recipes that are marked with a "V". You will then need to check the calorie count for each recipe to make sure you aren't exceeding the recommended 1,500 kcal a day.

On the evening before you begin, go for a good walk outside so you can make sure to sleep well.

THE LOW-CARB HIGH-FAT KITCHEN

Good fats, meat, fish, vegetables, fruit, salads, and dairy products—eating generously in all these categories will enhance the LCHF diet. The only area where you need to be careful is with foods that are rich in carbohydrates. So, clean out your store cupboard and refrigerator to remove any carb temptation. Make a shopping list for the first week's meals so you have everything to hand at home. And remember that buying fresh, organic produce where possible will create the healthiest and tastiest meals. As your food portions will be controlled, be generous with the quality of the ingredients.

FATS AND OILS
avocado, hemp, coconut, linseed, olive oil
beef tallow, animal fats (goose fat, duck fat, lard)
butter, ghee, clarified butter
nut oils (walnut, hazelnut, macadamia nut oil)

FISH AND SHELLFISH
eel, herring, salmon, mackerel
mussels
preserved in olive oil (sardines, tuna)
shrimp, crab

MEAT AND MEAT PRODUCTS
lamb, beef, pork, game
offal (liver, kidney)
poultry, skin on (chicken, duck, goose, turkey)
rich bone broth
salami, chorizo, ham, bacon

MILK PRODUCTS
cream, quark
high-fat cheese
sheep cheese (feta)

NUTS AND SEEDS
almonds, brazil nuts, pecans, macadamia
chia seeds, flaxseed, linseed

VEGETABLES AND SALAD
all varieties of cabbage, sauerkraut
all varieties of lettuce
asparagus (green and white)
artichoke
avocado
bell peppers
celery, cucumber, radish
eggplant, zucchini
olives
mushrooms
scallions, leek
Swiss chard, spinach
tomatoes

FRUIT
apples
apricots, plums
berries
grapefruit, oranges
lychee, papaya
pomegranate

HERBS, SPICES, SEASONINGS
all kinds of herbs
mayonnaise, aioli, béarnaise sauce
pesto
sugar-free mustard (mustard powder)
tomato purée

OTHER
eggs
dark chocolate (at least 80% cocoa solids)

USEFUL STORECUPBOARD ADDITIONS

It's recommended you stock up on the ingredients below before you begin the 28-day LCHF plan. While some of these ingredients may sound unusual, they should all be available at your local health food store. If you don't have them to hand, please feel free to substitute any of the specialist ingredients mentioned with locally sourced alternatives.

ACID-BASE POWDER

Ketones are acids and they accumulate in greater quantities on a LCHF diet. To keep the acid-alkaline balance in equilibrium while maintaining ketosis, an additional alkaline supplement is required. The best approach is to use an alkaline powder based on citrates, which offers protection against acidosis. These supplements are available from drugstores or online.

AJVAR

This red bell pepper paste originates from the Balkans. Combining garlic, eggplant, red bell peppers and olive oil, it makes a delicious, low-carb condiment, provided you buy (or make) a version without too much sugar—it's best to substitute stevia instead. Ajvar is available at major supermarkets and online. You can also substitute it with sun-dried tomato.

ALMOND FLOUR

After the almonds are pressed in an oil mill, the resulting cake is finely ground, then sold as partially de-oiled almond flour. This is very low in carbohydrates and so is an ideal replacement for traditional cereal flours. The flour is also available with its natural fat content. For the recipes in this book we have used partially de-oiled almond flour. You will find it in organic and health food stores.

BIRCH SUGAR (XYLITOL)

Birch sugar, also known as xylitol, is a natural sweetener. It originally comes from birch bark but nowadays is usually manufactured synthetically. It tastes very similar to household sugar but is much more expensive. In return, however, it increases blood sugar levels significantly less than traditional sugar because only 25 percent of its carbohydrates are broken down. Birch sugar is a good LCHF-compatible alternative to cane sugar. 1 teaspoon contains 1 kcal and no significant carbohydrate content.

CHIA SEEDS

The content of omega-3 fatty acids in chia seeds is unrivaled. They also contain large quantities of iron, magnesium, calcium, vitamins, and fiber. So these little, gluten-free seeds are justifiably regarded as a superfood. They also swell easily, which makes them great as a binding agent and for baking.

COCONUT FLOUR

The flour is produced from the dried, partially de-oiled flesh of the coconut which is then ground. It is gluten-free and its sweet coconut flavor can be used to enhance lots of dishes—either sweet or savory. Its absorbent properties also make it ideal for thickening sauces.

COCONUT OIL

Coconut oil is particularly good for frying because it is very stable when exposed to heat. It is also great for baking. When purchasing, look for the virgin organic product. Don't confuse coconut oil with solidified coconut fat. The subtle coconut flavor of the oil gives dishes a delicate hint of coconut. If you are not so keen on the taste, instead of using the virgin oil seek out a so-called deodorized variety, where the flavorings have been removed. Coconut oil (including flavorless varieties) can be found in organic stores, health food stores, and from online retailers.

COCONUT SUGAR

This sugar is ideal for the LCHF diet thanks to the minimal impact it has on blood sugar levels. It is produced from the sap of the coconut flower, which is exuded when the flower is cut.

The sugar crystals form as the substance undergoes evaporation. It can be used just like traditional sugar, it is roughly equivalent in sweetness to household sugar. It has a slightly caramel-like flavor but does not taste of coconut. 1 teaspoon of coconut sugar contains 19 kcal and 5 g carbohydrates.

CREAMED COCONUT

The finely grated white flesh of the coconut contains lots of oil and plant protein but few carbohydrates. It adds flavor and texture to sweet and savory dishes. Like coconut oil, you will find it in the supermarket, at drugstores, or from organic retailers. It's important to look for organic varieties here, too.

ERYTHRITOL

If a bit of sweetness is essential, this artificial sweetener is tolerated better than many other sweeteners. Erythritol contains almost no calories or carbohydrates. It is also found naturally in cheese, fruit, and pistachios.

GROUND PSYLLIUM HUSKS

The finely ground husks of the psyllium seed are used as a binding and swelling agent. The powder made from the husks of the psyllium plant has practically no carbohydrates and consists of over 80 percent dietary fiber. The recipes in this book exclusively use ready-ground psyllium husks. Substituting the same quantity of coarsely ground psyllium seed husks will not produce the same result. You can get the powder at health food stores and from organic retailers.

KETONE TEST STRIPS

These strips for measuring ketosis levels in the urine can be bought at drugstores. They are simply dipped into the urine. Ketone levels can be determined very simply by comparing the change in color to a comparison scale, which allows you to infer your blood ketone levels.

LICORICE POWDER

The sap of the licorice root is tapped and dried, then finely ground to produce licorice powder.

The powder is perfect for flavoring sweet or savory dishes. You will find it at drugstores, health food stores, or online. Some people experience high blood pressure in response to licorice. Anyone affected should speak to their physician before using it.

QUARK

A kind of curd without the added rennet or salt, quark originates from Eastern Europe. It is a soft white cheese typically described as a cross between yogurt and cottage cheese, made by warming soured milk until it curdles. It is ideal for the LCHF diet as it is high in protein (14 g per 100g) and can be high in fat (up to 40%) with negligible carbs. You can find quark online or at organic grocery and health food stores, or you can make your own.

SESAME SEED FLOUR

To make sesame seed flour, unroasted sesame seeds are de-oiled, then finely ground. It has a relatively neutral flavor and so is ideal as a flour substitute in baking. It only contains approx. 6 g carbohydrates for each 100 g (roughly equivalent to ¼ ounce per 4 ounces) and is ideal for LCHF cuisine. It can be sourced online.

STEVIA

Available in liquid or crystalline form, this extract obtained from the stevia plant is several hundred times sweeter than ordinary sugar. Due to its bitter, licorice-like aftertaste, stevia is not to everyone's liking. But it is great for a LCHF diet because it contains no calories and doesn't impact your blood sugar levels.

VANILLA POWDER

Not to be confused with vanilla sugar. To make vanilla powder the entire dried pod is finely ground. The powder is many times more intense than vanilla sugar and, most importantly, it is free from artificial additives and sugar. You will find it at drugstores, organic groceries, and health food stores.

WEEK 1

The recipes below are carefully planned to provide you with 1,500 calories a day. As each recipe indicates the calories, you may substitute for a similar recipe. Remember to cut out the sodas and too much caffeine and drink plenty of water, at least two large bottles a day. Weigh yourself to start and measure the ketone levels every morning (see page 21).

(see page 21)

	BREAKFAST	LUNCH	SNACK/SWEET	DINNER
MONDAY	Waffles with raspberry quark-style cheese (p.40)	Zucchini omelet with Serrano ham (p.82)	Lemon and yogurt gelées (p.160)	Chicken in buttermilk sauce (p.150) 105
TUESDAY	Almond pancakes with sour cherry compote (p.42)	Chicken nuggets with baked tomatoes (p.84)	"Quattro formaggi" muffins (p.148)	Lemon shrimp on creamed spinach (p.129)
WEDNESDAY	Quark flatbread with chocolate spread (p.44)	Moussaka (p.76)	Almond and coconut cookies (p.168)	Chicken legs in bacon sauce with Savoy cabbage (p.114)
THURSDAY	White coffee smoothie (p.46)	Cheese tortillas with guacamole (p.73)	Mini bell peppers with cream cheese (p.152)	Meatballs with asparagus salad (p.104)
FRIDAY	Salami omelet (p.48)	Tomato and red bell pepper soup with Parmesan chips (p.86)	Peanut bars (p.166)	Sea bream on green asparagus (p.130)
SATURDAY	Crunchy nut muesli (p.59)	Cheese tortillas with guacamole (p.73)	Avocado and chocolate muffins (p.163)	Pork medallions with a tomato and pepper medley (p.100)
SUNDAY	Avocado with smoked salmon mousse (p.56)	Beef soup (p.96)	Crispy zucchini with herb aioli (p.146)	Ribeye steak with sauerkraut and creamy cabbage (p.117)

WEEK 2

There is a new menu of delicious recipes for you this week. The desire for carbs and sweet things can be powerful. This craving does gradually diminish, but if all else fails, you can start with adding suitable sweeteners to your food. Try gradually to reduce your reliance on sweeteners; instead reward yourself with an occasional chunk of dark chocolate. It's time for a weigh in, but don't worry if you don't see much change yet.

	BREAKFAST	LUNCH	SNACK/SWEET	DINNER
MONDAY	Quark flatbread with chocolate spread (p.44)	Marinated tray-roasted summer vegetables with meatballs (p.70)	Egg carpaccio with dip (p.143)	Chicken curry with stuffed mushrooms (p.108)
TUESDAY	Bacon and quark tarte flambée (p.54)	Tuna fishcakes with cucumber salad (p.69)	Chocolate coconut balls (p.165)	Zucchini lasagna with soy bolognese (p.102)
WEDNESDAY	Crackers with radish and cottage cheese (p.55)	Souvlaki kebabs with marinated feta (p.74)	Mini eggplant pizzas (p.138)	Marinated pork neck steaks with star anise (p.116)
THURSDAY	Avocado smoothie with cardamom (p.47)	Chicken nuggets with baked tomatoes (p.84)	Avocado and chocolate muffins (p.163)	Chicken in buttermilk sauce (p.105)
FRIDAY	Almond pancakes with sour cherry compote (p.42)	Cauliflower and spinach bake (p.91)	Peanut bars (p.166)	Redfish on zucchini noodles (p.133)
SATURDAY	Salmon pancakes with scallion dip (p.57)	Beef soup (p.96)	Mini bell peppers with cream cheese (p.152)	Pork tenderloin in mustard sauce with Savoy cabbage and mushrooms (p.113)
SUNDAY	Waffles with raspberry quark-style cheese (p.40)	Sauerkraut and bacon patties (p.90)	Almond and coconut cookies (p.168)	Duck breast on a bed of chicory (p.123)

WEEK 3

By now your cravings should have diminished, so you can look to increase your exercise and activity. A good daily walk is a minimum, but pick up the pace if you can with something you enjoy—yoga, swimming, or cycling are all good. You should see a weight reduction by now. Remember to keep up the fluid intake.

	BREAKFAST	LUNCH	SNACK/SWEET	DINNER
MONDAY	Crunchy nut muesli (p.59)	Zucchini omelet with Serrano ham (p.82)	Eggs baked in tomatoes (p.143)	Halloumi with a papaya and tomato salsa (p.124)
TUESDAY	Avocado with smoked salmon mousse (p.56)	Veggie spaghetti with mushroom sauce (p.88)	Parmesan and zucchini patties with red pesto (p.141)	Monkfish in an orange and pepper sauce (p.134)
WEDNESDAY	Salami omelet (p.48)	Chicken nuggets with baked tomatoes (p.84)	Almond and coconut cookies (p.168)	Meatballs with asparagus salad (p.104)
THURSDAY	Cream cheese smoothie with strawberries (p.46)	Sauerkraut and bacon patties (p.90)	Spinach muffins with bacon (p.150)	Pork medallions with a tomato and pepper medley (p.100)
FRIDAY	Coconut pancakes with blueberry yogurt (p.43)	Tuna fishcakes with cucumber salad (p.69)	Yogurt panna cotta with strawberry sauce (p.157)	Zucchini lasagna with soy bolognese (p.102)
SATURDAY	Waffles with raspberry quark-style cheese (p.40)	Souvlaki kebabs with marinated feta (p.74)	Crispy zuccini with herb aioli (p.146)	Ribeye steak with sauerkraut and creamy cabbage (p.117)
SUNDAY	Cottage cheese flatbread (p.61)	Moussaka (p.76)	"Quattro formaggi" muffins (p.148)	Lamb fillet with a parsley and mustard topping (p.110)

WEEK 4

Well done for making it to the last week. You should be feeling lighter, more energized, and more focused. You don't need to stop the diet after this week. Now you have the recipes under your belt and plenty more in the book to explore, go ahead and enjoy cooking and eating more LCHF meals.

	BREAKFAST	LUNCH	SNACK/SWEET	DINNER
MONDAY	Almond pancakes with sour cherry compote (p.42)	Cheese tortillas with guacamole (p.82)	Stuffed eggs with bacon (p.142)	Marinated pork neck steaks with star anise (p.116)
TUESDAY	Quark flatbread with chocolate spread (p.44)	Marinated tray-roasted summer vegetables with meatballs (p.70)	Lemon and yogurt gelées (p.160)	Cauliflower risotto (p.126)
WEDNESDAY	Salmon pancakes with scallion dip (p.57)	Cauliflower and spinach bake (p.91)	Peanut bars (p.166)	Chicken curry with stuffed mushrooms (p.108)
THURSDAY	Blueberry and licorice smoothie (p.47)	Tomato and red bell pepper soup with Parmesan chips (p.152)	Chocolate coconut balls (p.165)	Chicken in buttermilk sauce (p.105)
FRIDAY	Waffles with raspberry quark-style cheese (p.41)	Moussaka (p.76)	Parmesan and zucchini patties with red pesto (p.141)	Lemon shrimp on creamed spinach (p.129)
SATURDAY	Crunchy nut muesli (p.59)	Chicken nuggets with baked tomatoes (p.84)	Mini eggplant pizzas (p.138)	Lamb fillet with a parsley and mustard topping (p.110)
SUNDAY	Bacon and quark tarte flambée (p.54)	Cauliflower and turmeric cheese fritters (p.85)	Choco-nut bites (p.164)	Pork tenderloin in mustard sauce with Savoy cabbage and mushrooms (p.113)

2

BREAKFAST

Sweet or savory is not so important,
but getting the day off to a keto start is
crucial. Try simple standbys or quick russle
ups, like scrambled eggs or fruit salad.
To make sure you have time for a substantial
breakfast, lots of the preparation can be
done the night before.

ORANGE AND CHIA
CREAM WITH PISTACHIOS

zest and juice of 1 orange

3 medium eggs

scant ½ cup (100 g) cream

1 tablespoon chia seeds, plus extra for
    scattering

1⅓ cup (100 g) shelled pistachios
    (roasted, unsalted)

Serves 2

Preparation: approx. 20 minutes

Per portion: approx. 480 kcal, 19 g
protein, 39 g fat, 10 g carbohydrate

Choose a pan that is large enough to form a bain-marie, fill with
½ inch (1 cm) water, and bring to a boil.

Meanwhile, measure a scant 100 ml/½ cup of the orange
juice and mix this with the orange zest, eggs and cream in a
heatproof bowl (metal, if possible) until smooth. Heat the mixture
over the bain-marie, stirring constantly, for 5–6 minutes until it
has thickened.

Stir in the chia seeds and stand the bowl in cold water to chill
for 10 minutes to prevent it cooking any further. Stir the cream
occasionally as it cools.

Divide the cream between two little bowls and serve scattered
with pistachios and chia seeds.

PREPARE THE NIGHT BEFORE

This creamy dish is great prepared ahead of time. In fact, after
chilling overnight in the refrigerator the consistency will be even
creamier. The following morning, just scatter over the pistachios
and chia seeds, and it's ready to enjoy.

WAFFLES WITH
RASPBERRY QUARK-STYLE CHEESE

FOR THE WAFFLES
3 medium eggs
$^1/_3$ cup (75 g) cream
3 tablespoons ground psyllium husks
salt
soft butter, for greasing

FOR THE QUARK
scant ½ cup (50 g) raspberries, plus
    extra to serve
heaping ¾ cup (200 g) quark
    (40% fat)
3 tablespoons Greek yogurt

Serves: 2
Preparation: approx. 25 minutes
Per portion: approx. 435 kcal, 23 g
protein, 34 g fat, 7 g carbohydrate

Stir the eggs, cream, ground psyllium husks, a pinch of salt, and $^2/_3$ cup (150 ml) cold water with a whisk until you have a smooth batter. Leave the batter to stand for 5 minutes.

Meanwhile, crush them slightly in a bowl using a fork. Add the quark and yogurt and stir together until creamy.

Heat the waffle iron to medium, then use a pastry brush to apply a thin layer of butter over the surface. Put a quarter of the batter into the waffle maker, close, and cook for 3–4 minutes until light golden brown and crisp. Transfer to a plate, cover and keep warm. Make three more waffles in the same way with the remaining batter. Arrange on two plates and serve with the quark and a few extra raspberries.

NO WAFFLE MAKER?

No worries, the batter can also be used to make pancakes. To do this, melt 1 tablespoon butter in a large, non-stick pan over medium heat. For one small pancake, add 1 tablespoon of batter and cook for 2 minutes, then flip it over using a spatula and cook for 2 minutes on the other side. The batter will make roughly eight small pancakes, which go just as well with the raspberry quark as the waffles.

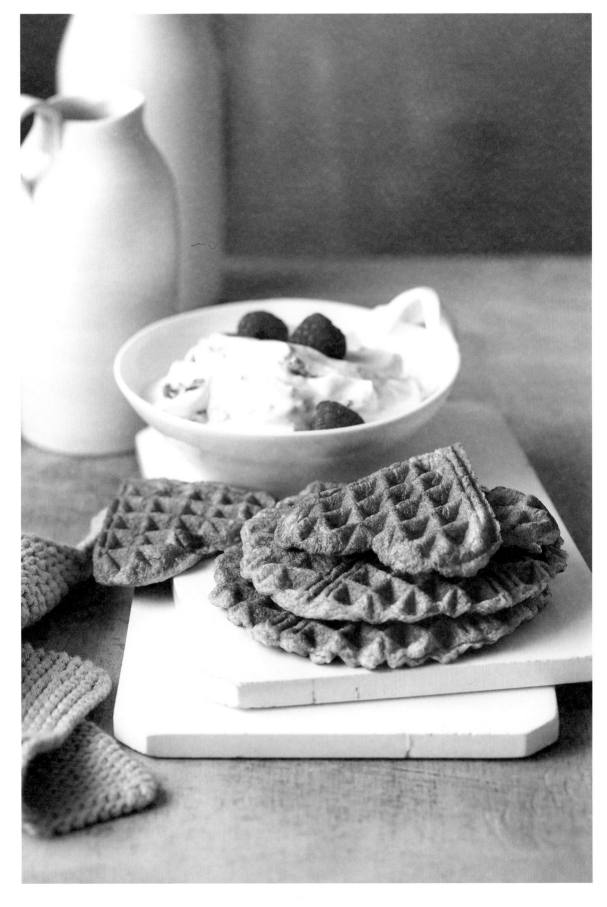

ALMOND PANCAKES
WITH SOUR CHERRY COMPOTE

(V)

FOR THE PANCAKES
3 medium eggs
¼ cup (50 g) cream
1 tablespoon almond butter
½ cup (50 g) ground almonds
1 tablespoon ground psyllium husks
½ teaspoon vanilla powder
3 tablespoons coconut oil

FOR THE COMPOTE
⅔ cup (100 g) sour cherries (or defrosted
    frozen sour cherries)
1 tablespoon lemon juice
½ teaspoon ground cardamom
½ teaspoon ground cinnamon
1 tablespoon chia seeds

Serves: 2
Preparation: approx. 15 minutes
Standing time: approx. 10 minutes
Per portion: approx. 600 kcal, 19 g
protein, 53 g fat, 10 g carbohydrate

To make the pancakes, put the eggs, cream, almond butter, ground almonds, ground psyllium husks, and vanilla powder into a bowl with scant ½ cup (100 ml) water and whisk swiftly to create a smooth batter. Let the batter sit for 10 minutes.

Meanwhile, wash and pit the sour cherries, removing any stems. Put the cherries into a pan with the lemon juice and 1 tablespoon of water, bring briefly to a boil, then remove from the heat. Stir in the cardamom, cinnamon, and chia seeds and let sit for about 10 minutes.

Heat the coconut oil in a large non-stick frying pan. Add 1–2 tablespoons of batter to the pan for each pancake and cook over medium heat for 1–2 minutes until golden brown underneath. Flip over and continue cooking on the other side for 1–2 minutes until golden.

Make a total of eight pancakes, arrange on two plates, and serve with the cherry compote.

COCONUT PANCAKES
WITH BLUEBERRY YOGURT

FOR THE PANCAKES

3 medium eggs
$^1/_3$ cup (80 g) crème fraîche
2 tablespoons desiccated coconut
2 teaspoons ground psyllium husks
3 tablespoons coconut oil

FOR THE YOGURT

$^1/_3$ cup (50 g) blueberries
1½ cups (200 g) yogurt
1 tablespoon creamed coconut
½ teaspoon vanilla powder
birch sugar (xylitol), optional

Serves: 2
Preparation: approx. 25 minutes
Standing time: approx. 10 minutes
Per portion: approx. 635 kcal, 16 g
protein, 59 g fat, 9 g carbohydrate

Briskly whisk the eggs, crème fraîche, desiccated coconut, and ground psyllium husks to create a smooth batter. Let sit for about 10 minutes.

Meanwhile, mash the blueberries slightly with a fork. Add the yogurt, creamed coconut, and vanilla powder and stir. If desired, adjust to taste with some birch sugar. Transfer to the fridge.

Heat the coconut oil in a large non-stick frying pan. Use 1–2 tablespoons of batter per pancake and cook, covered, over medium heat for roughly 2 minutes until golden brown. Flip them over and continue cooking on the other side for 1–2 minutes until golden.

Make a total of eight pancakes, arrange them between two plates, and serve with the blueberry yogurt.

WARM OR COLD

Everyone has their own preference. These pancakes can easily be prepared the previous evening and still taste great cold the following morning. If that doesn't appeal, you can either cook them fresh in the morning or briefly reheat them in the microwave or oven.

QUARK FLATBREAD
WITH CHOCOLATE SPREAD

(V)

FOR THE QUARK FLATBREADS

¹/₃ cup (100 g) quark
     (40% fat)
2 medium eggs, separated
2 tablespoons almond flour
1 teaspoon ground psyllium husks
salt

FOR THE CHOCOLATE SPREAD

1 avocado
1 tablespoon cream
1 tablespoon cocoa powder
birch sugar (xylitol), optional

Serves 2
Preparation: approx. 20 minutes
Baking: approx. 30 minutes
Per portion: approx. 475 kcal, 25 g
protein, 39 g fat, 4 g carbohydrate

Preheat the oven to 300°F (150°C). Line a baking tray with parchment paper. Squeeze the quark thoroughly in a clean dish towel to remove as much moisture as possible. Whisk the egg whites with a pinch of salt until stiff. Quickly stir together the quark, egg yolks, almond flour and ground psyllium husks. Carefully fold in the whisked egg whites.

Use a tablespoon to create four equal dollops of quark mixture on the baking tray, and press slightly flat. Bake in the center of the oven for 25–30 minutes. Turn off the oven and allow the breads to cool inside. Let cool in the oven.

Meanwhile, prepare the chocolate spread. To do this, halve the avocado, remove the pit, and scoop out the flesh. Transfer to a blender along with the cream, cocoa powder, and, if desired, the birch sugar. Blend to a purée.

Serve the cooled quark flatbreads on two plates, topped with the chocolate spread.

QUARK ROLLS

These protein-rich, quark flatbreads also make a great alternative to bread rolls. Since they have neither a sweet nor savory flavor themselves, they taste just as delicious with slightly sweet toppings and spreads (such as the chocolate spread here) or with savory toppings, such as a slice of sausage or cheese.

WHITE COFFEE SMOOTHIE

²/₃ cup (150 ml) cold coffee
²/₃ cup (150 ml) almond milk
    (unsweetened)
¹/₃ cup (100 g) sour cream
¹/₃ cup (50 g) blanched almonds
1 tablespoon creamed coconut
3 medium eggs
½ teaspoon vanilla powder
birch sugar (xylitol), optional
4 ice cubes
cocoa powder, for decorating

Serves 2
Preparation: approx. 10 minutes
Per portion: approx. 490 kcal, 18 g
protein, 43 g fat, 9 g carbohydrate

Put the coffee into a blender along with the almond milk, sour cream, almonds, creamed coconut, eggs, and vanilla powder. Blend until the almonds are finely ground and all the ingredients are thoroughly combined. If desired, adjust to taste with some birch sugar.

Add two ice cubes each to two large glasses and pour over the coffee smoothie. Top with a dusting of cocoa powder and serve immediately.

NOTE

Eating raw eggs can pose a health risk, especially to the elderly, young children under the age of four, pregnant women, and other highly susceptible individuals with compromised immune systems. Make sure that foods that contain raw or lightly cooked eggs are made only with organic, pasteurized eggs. If desired, the eggs in these recipes can be removed.

CREAM CHEESE SMOOTHIE WITH STRAWBERRIES

1 cup (150 g) strawberries, hulled
heaping ½ cup (140 g) full-fat
    cream cheese
¾ cup (180 g) coconut milk (canned)
2 medium eggs
½ teaspoon vanilla powder
birch sugar (xylitol), optional

Serves 2
Preparation: approx. 15 minutes
Per portion: approx. 465 kcal,
14 g protein, 41 g fat, 8 g carbohydrate

Depending on how large they are, slice the strawberries into halves or quarters. Set aside four strawberry halves for decoration.

Put the remaining strawberries into a blender with the cream cheese, coconut milk, eggs, and vanilla powder and blend until smooth. If desired, adjust to taste with some birch sugar.

Pour the smoothie into two large glasses, decorate with the halved strawberries, and serve.

NOTE

Eating raw eggs can pose a health risk, especially to the elderly, young children under the age of four, pregnant women, and other highly susceptible individuals with compromised immune systems. Make sure that foods that contain raw or lightly cooked eggs are made only with organic, pasteurized eggs. If desired, the eggs in these recipes can be removed.

AVOCADO SMOOTHIE
WITH CARDAMOM

1 avocado, halved and pitted
2 medium eggs
scant ½ cup (100 g) coconut milk
    (canned)
¼ cup (50 g) cream
½ teaspoon vanilla powder
½ teaspoon ground cardamom
¾ cup (100 g) raspberries
birch sugar (xylitol), optional
6 ice cubes

Serves 2
Preparation: approx. 15 minutes
Per portion: approx. 525 kcal,
12 g protein, 50 g fat, 5 g carbohydrate

Put the avocado flesh into a blender and add the eggs, coconut milk, cream, vanilla powder, cardamom, and raspberries (reserving four of the best for decoration) and blend until smooth. Add ½–⅓ cup (100–150 ml) water depending on the desired consistency and purée the smoothie again. If desired, adjust to taste with some birch sugar.

Put three ice cubes each into two large glasses and pour over the smoothie. Decorate with the reserved raspberries and serve.

NOTE
Eating raw eggs can pose a health risk, especially to the elderly, young children under the age of four, pregnant women, and other highly susceptible individuals with compromised immune systems. Make sure that foods that contain raw or lightly cooked eggs are made only with organic, pasteurized eggs. If desired, the eggs in these recipes can be removed.

BLUEBERRY AND
LICORICE SMOOTHIE

1 cup (150 g) blueberries
1¼ cup (300 g) sour cream
½ cup (150 g) Greek yogurt
3 tablespoons creamed coconut
1 teaspoon licorice powder
1 teaspoon vanilla powder
birch sugar (xylitol), optional

Serves 2
Preparation: approx. 10 minutes
Per portion: approx. 630 kcal,
9 g protein, 58 g fat, 16 g carbohydrate

Set aside four of the best blueberries for decoration.

Add the remaining blueberries to a blender along with the sour cream, yogurt, creamed coconut, licorice powder, and vanilla powder and purée until smooth. If desired, adjust to taste with some birch sugar.

Transfer into two large glasses, decorate with the reserved blueberries and serve.

SALAMI OMELET

1¾ oz (50 g) Gouda (or other hard
    cheese), roughly grated
1¾ oz (50 g) Parmesan, roughly grated
3 medium eggs
2 tablespoons cream
2 teaspoons butter
4 chives, cut into little pieces
6 slices of salami
2 sprigs of cilantro
salt and pepper

Serves 2
Preparation: approx. 25 minutes
Per portion: approx. 400 kcal,
29 g protein, 31 g fat, 1 g carbohydrate

Mix the Gouda and Parmesan. Beat the eggs and cream with a
fork and season with salt and pepper.

Melt 1 teaspoon butter in a non-stick pan over medium heat.
Spread half the cheese mixture evenly over the pan, cover, and
let the cheese melt for 1 minute.

Add half the egg mixture over the cheese, distributing it evenly
by swirling the pan. Cover the pan and cook the egg mixture
over medium heat for 2 minutes. Wash and shake dry the chives
and snip into little pieces.

Cover one half of the omelet with three slices of salami and carefully fold over the other half of the omelet using a spatula. Cover
the pan again and continue cooking the omelet for 2 minutes.
Flip the omelet and cook the other side for another 2 minutes
until the egg mixture has completely set.

Slip the omelet onto a plate and cover with aluminum foil to keep
warm. Cook a second omelet from the remaining ingredients.
Scatter chopped chives over both omelets and garnish with
cilantro to serve.

A RANGE OF FILLINGS

Use these ingredients as fillings to ensure you get plenty of
variety at the breakfast table: different hard cheeses such as
Monterey Jack or Edam, which give similar results to Gouda;
finely chopped vegetables such as cherry tomatoes, shallots, red
onions, or bell pepper. Add in some aromatic fresh herbs such
as basil, oregano, flat-leaf parsley, thyme, or sage. Have you
got some leftover smoked ham lurking in your refrigerator? Or
maybe some Parma ham or smoked turkey breast or even some
bacon? Fantastic, just toss it into the omelet!

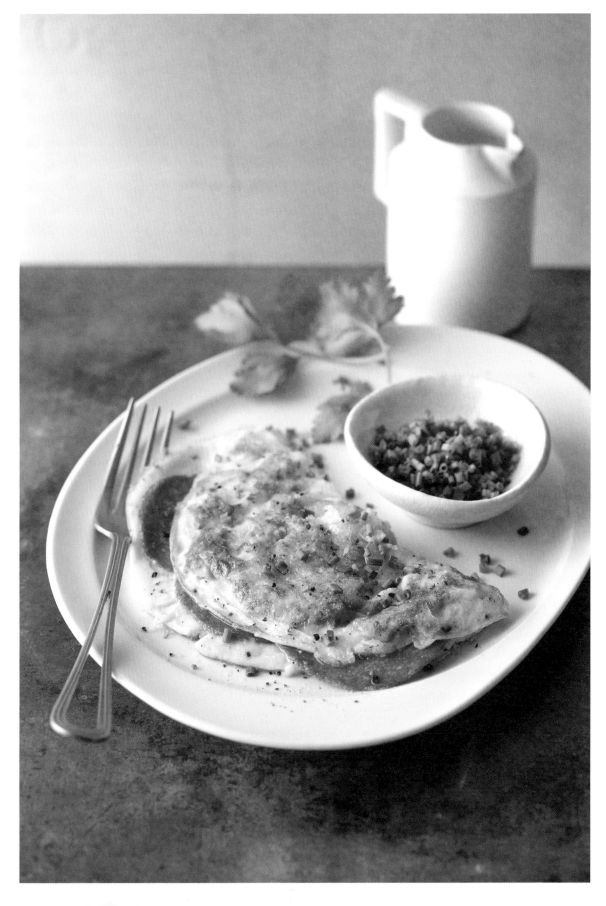

GOUDA, TOMATO, AND HAM OMELET

4 medium eggs
2½ tablespoons cream
8 teaspoons butter
2 tomatoes, cut into roughly 5-mm
    (¼ inch) thick slices
1½ oz (40 g) Gouda, roughly grated
2 slices of cooked ham, finely chopped
salt and pepper

Serves 2
Preparation: approx. 15 minutes
Per portion: approx. 495 kcal,
31 g protein, 40 g fat, 3 g carbohydrate

Whisk the eggs into the cream until smooth and season with salt and pepper. Melt 4 teaspoons butter in a non-stick pan over medium heat. Add half the egg mixture and tilt the pan to distribute evenly. Cover the pan and cook the egg mixture for 2 minutes.

Cover one half of the omelet with half the sliced tomato, cheese, and ham. Carefully fold over the other half of the omelet using a spatula. Return the lid to the pan and continue cooking for 1 minute. Turn the omelet and cook the other side for 1 minute, until the egg mixture has set completely and the cheese inside has melted.

Slide the filled omelet onto a plate and cover with aluminum foil to keep warm. Make a second omelet in the same way from the remaining ingredients and serve.

SPINACH AND BLUE CHEESE OMELET

²/₃ cup (150 g) fresh spinach
   (or 5 oz frozen)
4 medium eggs
2½ tablespoons cream
freshly grated nutmeg
2 teaspoons butter
3 oz (80 g) blue cheese
salt and pepper

Serves 2
Preparation: approx. 15 minutes
Per portion: approx. 435 kcal,
21 g protein, 38 g fat, 2 g carbohydrate

Carefully wash the fresh spinach and let drain (or defrost the frozen spinach according to the instructions on the pack, let drain in a sieve and squeeze out well). Add the spinach to a blender with the eggs, cream, salt, pepper, and nutmeg and blend until smooth.

Melt 1 teaspoon of butter in a non-stick pan over medium heat. Add half the egg mixture and tilt the pan to distribute evenly. Cover the pan and cook the egg mixture for 2 minutes.

Crumble half the blue cheese over one half of the omelet. Carefully fold over the other half of the omelet using a spatula, cover, and continue cooking for 1 minute. Flip the omelet over, cover, and cook the other side for 1 minute until the spinach mixture has set and the cheese inside has melted.

Slip the omelet onto a plate and cover with aluminum foil to keep warm. Make the second omelet in the same way from the remaining ingredients and serve.

OVEN-BAKED OMELET WITH CREAMED MUSHROOMS

4 medium eggs
²/₃ cup (150 g) cream
3 sprigs of parsley, finely chopped
freshly grated nutmeg
1 teaspoon butter
2 ¾ cups (150 g) chanterelles (or other mushrooms), large ones halved or quartered
3 slices of cooked ham, diced
salt and pepper

Serves 2
Preparation: approx. 20 minutes
Per portion: approx. 455 kcal,
23 g protein, 39 g fat, 3 g carbohydrate

Line a high-sided baking tray up to the rim with parchment paper. Preheat the oven to 400°F (200°C).

Whisk together the eggs, a scant ½ cup (100 g) of the cream, and the chopped parsley until smooth. Season with salt, pepper, and nutmeg. Pour the egg mixture over the baking tray and tilt the tray to spread it out evenly. Place the tray in the center of the oven and bake for 10 minutes until the egg mixture has set completely and has started to brown slightly.

Meanwhile, melt the butter in a pan over a high heat and sauté the mushrooms for 2 minutes. Add the diced ham and continue cooking everything for a further 1 minute.

Pour in the remaining cream, bring to a boil, and simmer for 1 minute until it has reduced to a thick and creamy sauce. Season to taste with more salt, pepper, and nutmeg.

Remove the omelet from the oven and use the parchment paper to transfer it to a chopping board. Use a spatula to help release it from the parchment paper and roll it up. Slice diagonally into six equal pieces, transfer onto two plates, and serve with the creamy chanterelle mushrooms.

MIX IT UP

You can use other types of mushroom instead of the chanterelles. Button mushrooms, king oyster mushrooms, shiitake, and Chinese mushrooms are available all year round. Or maybe you've gone out mushroom picking and gathered a good haul yourself; in which case, you can use this recipe to rustle up something truly delicious from your basket.

BACON AND
QUARK TARTE FLAMBÉE

¹/₃ cup (100 g) quark (20% fat)
2 medium eggs
1 tablespoon coconut flour
5 oz (150 g) Gouda, roughly grated
2 scallions, finely sliced
5 strips bacon, finely chopped
¹/₃ cup (80 g) crème fraîche
salt

Serves 2
Preparation: approx. 20 minutes
Baking: approx. 35 minutes
Per portion: approx. 585 kcal,
40 g protein, 45 g fat, 4 g carbohydrate

Preheat the oven to 350°F (170°C). Line a baking tray with parchment paper. Stir together the quark, eggs, coconut flour, a pinch of salt, and a third of the Gouda. Transfer to the baking tray and spread the mixture out to create a 7-inch (20 cm) square. Slide the tray into the center of the oven and bake for 15 minutes.

Remove the baking tray from the oven (but leave the oven on), spread the quark base with crème fraîche and scatter over the bacon, scallions, and remaining cheese.

Return to the oven to cook for a further 15–20 minutes until the cheese is nicely golden. Remove, slice into quarters, and serve on two plates.

A TASTY ALTERNATIVE

Try using red, yellow, or green bell peppers sliced into thin strips, little precooked broccoli florets, or sliced mushrooms.

CRACKERS WITH RADISH
AND COTTAGE CHEESE

(v)

FOR THE CRACKERS
½ cup (80 g) linseeds, whole
1 medium egg
1¾ oz (50 g) Gouda, roughly grated
1 tablespoon sesame seeds
1 tablespoon sunflower seeds
salt and pepper

FOR THE COTTAGE CHEESE
6 radishes, roughly grated
2 sprigs of fresh dill, leaves finely
    chopped
heaping ¾ cup (200 g) cottage cheese
    (curd cheese)
salt and pepper

Serves 2
Preparation: approx. 20 minutes
Baking: approx. 25 minutes
Per portion: approx. 485 kcal,
38 g protein, 31 g fat, 5 g carbohydrate

Whisk the linseeds into the egg and 2 tablespoons of lukewarm water then let sit for 15 minutes. Preheat the oven to 300°F (150°C). Line a baking tray with parchment paper.

Meanwhile, add the Gouda to the soaked linseed together with the sesame and sunflower seeds and stir well. Season with a pinch of salt and pepper.

Use a tablespoon to scoop eight equal-size portions of the mixture onto the baking tray, spacing them well apart. Press the dollops of mixture flat. Put the tray into the center of the oven and bake the crackers for a total of 25 minutes, turning once after 15 minutes.

Stir the radishes and dill into the cottage cheese and season to taste with salt and pepper.

Once the crackers are cooked, remove them from the oven and use the parchment paper to transfer them to a wire rack to cool completely. Arrange on two plates with the radish and cottage cheese to serve.

AVOCADO WITH SMOKED SALMON MOUSSE

5 oz (150 g) smoked salmon, chopped
    into small chunks
zest and juice of ½ lemon
¼ cup (50 g) full-fat cream cheese
⅓ cup (80 g) Greek yogurt
pinch of ground psyllium husks
4 sprigs of dill, leaves finely chopped
1 avocado, peeled and pitted
salt and pepper

Serves 2
Preparation: approx. 20 minutes
Per portion: approx. 490 kcal,
19 g protein, 44 g fat, 3 g carbohydrate

Put the salmon into a blender or food processor.

Add 1 tablespoon of the lemon juice with the lemon zest, cream cheese, yogurt, ground psyllium husks, and dill to the salmon and blend everything until smooth. Season to taste with salt and pepper. Chill the salmon mousse for 5 minutes.

Slice the avocado halves lengthwise into roughly ⅛-inch (4-mm) thick slices and arrange these in a fan pattern on two plates. Drizzle or brush the cut surfaces with the remaining lemon juice to prevent them from going brown.

Using a damp spoon, scoop up little mounds of salmon mousse and arrange these on the plates next to the avocado to serve.

SALMON PANCAKES
WITH SCALLION DIP

FOR THE PANCAKES
3½ oz (100 g) smoked salmon,
    roughly chopped
juice of ¼ lemon
2 medium eggs
2 tablespoons (30 g) cream
2 sprigs of dill, leaves picked
1 tablespoon ground psyllium husks
3 teaspoons coconut oil
salt and pepper

FOR THE DIP
3 scallions, sliced diagonally
1 tablespoon mayonnaise
¼ cup (50 g) sour cream
½ teaspoon mild ground paprika
salt and pepper

Serves 2
Preparation: approx. 25 minutes
Per portion: approx. 390 kcal,
18 g protein, 34 g fat, 3 g carbohydrate

Put the salmon, lemon juice, eggs, cream, and dill into a blender and process until smooth. Quickly fold in the ground psyllium husks, season to taste with salt and pepper, and let sit for 10 minutes.

Meanwhile, stir the scallions into the mayonnaise, sour cream, and ground paprika. Season to taste with salt and pepper.

Melt the coconut oil in a non-stick pan over medium heat. Make four pancakes, each using 1½ tablespoons of the mixture and cook each side in turn for 2–3 minutes. Transfer the salmon pancakes to a plate and serve with the dip.

CUCUMBER SALAD
Transform the dip into a cucumber salad, which also goes beautifully with the smoked salmon pancakes. Replace the scallion with ½ cucumber, peeled and thinly sliced, and add 1 tablespoon white wine vinegar: Your speedy cucumber salad is ready.

RICH ALMOND BREAD

coconut oil, for greasing
scant 1 cup (250 g) Greek yogurt
6 medium eggs
¼ cup (40 g) ground linseed
scant ½ cup (50 g) sunflower seeds
1¼ cup (120 g) ground almonds
2 tablespoons ground psyllium husks
2 teaspoons baking powder
salt

Makes 1 loaf (roughly 15 slices)
Preparation: approx. 15 minutes
Baking: approx. 45 minutes
Per slice: approx. 130 kcal, 6 g protein,
11 g fat, 2 g carbohydrate

Preheat the oven to 350°F (180°C). Grease a loaf tin with coconut oil. Mix the yogurt, eggs, and a pinch of salt in a bowl. Then add the linseed, sunflower seeds, and almonds and stir well.

Finally, add the ground psyllium husks and baking powder and fold in swiftly using a whisk. Leave the dough to rest for 10 minutes, then transfer to the greased loaf pan and bake in the center of the oven for 45 minutes.

Remove, let cool briefly, then carefully turn the bread out of the tin. Let cool completely on a wire rack.

SPICE IT UP

Give the loaf an unmistakable flavor and create endless different versions. Great options include fennel seeds, caraway, dried thyme, or rosemary. 1 teaspoon will suffice in each case. A dash of red wine vinegar gives the bread a pleasant acidity.

CRUNCHY NUT MUESLI

FOR THE MUESLI

2 tablespoons hazelnuts
1 tablespoon salted peanuts
1 tablespoon sliced almonds
1 tablespoon coconut flakes
1 tablespoon pumpkin seeds
1 tablespoon sunflower seeds
1 teaspoon coconut oil
pinch of ground cinnamon
½ teaspoon ground cardamom

FOR THE QUARK

heaping ¾ cup (200 g) quark
  (20% fat)
½ teaspoon vanilla powder
birch sugar (xylitol), optional

Serves 2
Preparation: approx. 15 minutes
Baking: approx. 10 minutes
Per portion: approx. 445 kcal, 22 g
protein, 36 g fat, 8 g carbohydrate

Preheat the oven to 325°F (160°C). Line a baking tray with parchment paper. Roughly chop the hazelnuts and peanuts. Add to a bowl with the sliced almonds, coconut flakes, pumpkin seeds, and sunflower seeds. Add the coconut oil, cinnamon, and cardamom and combine everything well using your hands.

Spread evenly over the baking tray and place in the center of the oven. Only bake as much in one go as will easily fit spread over the baking tray, otherwise you won't get a crunchy muesli. Bake for 8–10 minutes. Stir the mixture halfway through to ensure the nuts and seeds toast evenly.

Meanwhile, stir the quark and vanilla powder together until smooth. If desired, adjust to taste with some birch sugar. Divide the quark between two bowls. Remove the muesli from the oven, let cool slightly, sprinkle over the quark, and serve.

LINSEED CRISPBREADS

1 medium egg
²/₃ cup (100 g) ground linseed
2 tablespoons almond flour
salt

Makes 10
Preparation: approx. 15 minutes
Standing time: approx. 10 minutes
Baking: approx. 50 minutes
Per piece: approx. 65 kcal, 5 g protein,
4 g fat, 0 g carbohydrate

Put the egg into a blender with ¾ cup (200 ml) lukewarm water. Add the linseed, almond flour, and a pinch of salt and blitz until all the ingredients have come together. Let sit for about 10 minutes.

Line a baking tray with parchment paper. Spread the dough out on a baking tray using a dough scraper to create an ⅛-inch (3–4-mm) thick rectangle measuring roughly 12 × 11 inches (30 × 28 cm).

Slide the tray into the center of the oven, then switch the oven on to 275°F (140°C) and bake the crispbread for 50 minutes.

Remove and immediately slice into ten equal-sized pieces (roughly 2¹/₃ × 5½ inches/6 × 14 cm). Turn off the heat, return the tray to the oven, and leave the crispbread to cool completely with the door slightly ajar.

COTTAGE CHEESE FLATBREAD

8¾ oz (250 g) cottage cheese
   (curd cheese)
2 medium eggs
2 tablespoons sesame seed flour
1 tablespoon ground psyllium husks
2 teaspoons black and white
   sesame seeds
salt

Makes 1
Preparation: approx. 10 minutes
Standing time: approx. 10 minutes
Baking: approx. 25 minutes
Per piece: approx. 610 kcal, 58 g protein,
33 g fat, 16 g carbohydrate

Preheat the oven to 350°F (175°C). Line a baking tray with parchment paper.

Whisk together the cottage cheese, eggs, and a pinch of salt. Add the sesame seed flour and ground psyllium husks, whisk again, and let sit for 10 minutes.

Transfer the mixture to the center of the baking tray and use a dough scraper to shape it into a round flatbread measuring roughly ¾ inch (2 cm) thick and 7 inches (20 cm) in diameter.

Sprinkle with sesame seeds, slide the tray into the center of the oven and bake for 20–25 minutes. Remove from the oven, use the parchment paper to lift the flatbread from the tray, and let cool completely.

ADD HERB BUTTER TO GO WITH STEAK
Topped with a classic herb butter, this bread makes a fabulous accompaniment to grilled steak. To make this, finely chop the leaves from 1 sprig of tarragon, 2 sprigs of thyme, 3 sprigs of parsley, and ½ bunch of chervil. Snip 1 bunch of chives into little pieces, and peel and crush 1 clove of garlic. Mix everything into 5 ounces (150 g) soft butter and season to taste with salt and pepper. This will keep well in the refrigerator for 2 weeks.

3

LUNCH

You should feel refreshed and full of energy
after your lunch. These recipes are filling and
delicious, but they won't weigh you down.
Good planning is also part of good eating
and, in turn, good health. If you are short of
time, you can prepare something that night
before, then heat it up the next day to enjoy
at your leisure.

OVEN-BAKED SHRIMP WITH TOMATOES AND BUTTON MUSHROOMS

juice of ½ lemon

1 tablespoon harissa

1 garlic clove, finely chopped or crushed

5 tablespoons coconut oil

5 oz (150 g) raw frozen jumbo shrimp
(peeled, defrosted)

7 oz (200 g) cherry tomatoes

7 oz (200 g) button mushrooms, halved

1 small zucchini, cut into ⅛ in
(3 mm) dice

salt and pepper

Serves 2

Preparation: approx. 15 minutes

Cooking: approx. 15 minutes

Defrosting: approx. 2 hours

Per portion: approx. 335 kcal,
19 g protein, 27 g fat, 5 g C

Preheat the oven to 425°F (220°C). Line a baking tray with parchment paper.

Stir together the lemon juice, harissa, garlic, and coconut oil. Season to taste with salt and pepper and add the shrimp and vegetables. Mix everything thoroughly by hand and spread evenly over the baking tray. Bake for 12 minutes in the center of the oven. Arrange on two plates to serve.

TRY WITH PEPPER AND EGGPLANT

Use 3½ oz (100 g) finely diced yellow bell pepper in place of the cherry tomatoes and ½ small eggplant instead of the zucchini.

CURRY SOUP
WITH SHRIMP SKEWERS

8 raw frozen jumbo shrimp (peeled, defrosted)
3 tablespoons coconut oil
1 carrot, peeled and finely diced
½ red bell pepper, deseeded and finely diced
½ leek, finely diced
2 celery stalks, finely diced
1²/₃ cups (400 ml) vegetable stock
2 teaspoons curry powder
zest and juice of ½ lime
scant ½ cup (100 g) coconut milk (canned)
¼ cup (50 g) cream
salt and pepper

Serves 2
Preparation: approx. 25 minutes
Defrosting: approx. 2 hours
Per portion: approx. 335 kcal,
12 g protein, 28 g fat, 7 g carbohydrate

Soak two wooden skewers for 5 minutes to prevent them from burning. Spear four prawns on each skewer.

Heat 1 tablespoon of the coconut oil in a pan over medium heat and sauté the diced vegetables for 2 minutes. Add the vegetable stock and bring to a boil over high heat. Add the curry powder and simmer the soup over medium heat for about 8 minutes.

Stir the lime zest and juice, coconut milk, and cream into the soup and season to taste with salt and pepper. Don't cook the soup any more, just keep it warm.

Add the remaining coconut oil to a non-stick pan over high heat. Season the prawns with salt and pepper and sauté them for 1 minute on each side. Serve the soup in two deep bowls and garnish each with a prawn skewer.

MAKE YOUR OWN VEGETABLE BROTH

You can make your own vegetable broth by chopping up carrots, onions, potatoes, and a leek. Add aromatic herbs to taste. Drop into boiling water and simmer gently for 30 minutes, then strain and discard the vegetables keeping only the liquid.

SPICY CHICKEN AND BROCCOLI SOUP

4 teaspoons clarified butter
3½ oz (100 g) broccoli, florets halved or
    quartered
1¾ oz (50 g) button mushrooms,
    quartered
2 celery stalks, diced
1¼ cups (300 ml) chicken stock
5 oz (150 g) chicken breast, chopped into
    roughly ½ in (1 cm) cubes
1 mild red chili, finely sliced
¼ teaspoon mild paprika
½ teaspoon ground ginger
½ teaspoon ground turmeric
scant ½ cup (100 g) cream
2 tablespoons full-fat cream cheese
salt and pepper

Serves 2
Preparation: approx. 20 minutes
Per portion: approx. 435 kcal,
22 g protein, 36 g fat, 5 g carbohydrate

Heat the clarified butter in a pan over medium heat. Add the vegetables and sauté for 2 minutes. Pour over the chicken stock, add the chicken breast, and bring to a boil. Simmer, uncovered, over medium heat for about 10 minutes.

Add the chili, paprika, ginger, and turmeric. Stir in the cream and cream cheese, and don't allow the soup to boil again. Season to taste with salt and pepper, then serve in two deep bowls.

MAKE YOUR OWN CHICKEN STOCK

You can make your own chicken broth for the week by poaching a whole chicken slowly for 90 minutes. You can add chopped leek, celery, and carrot for extra flavor.

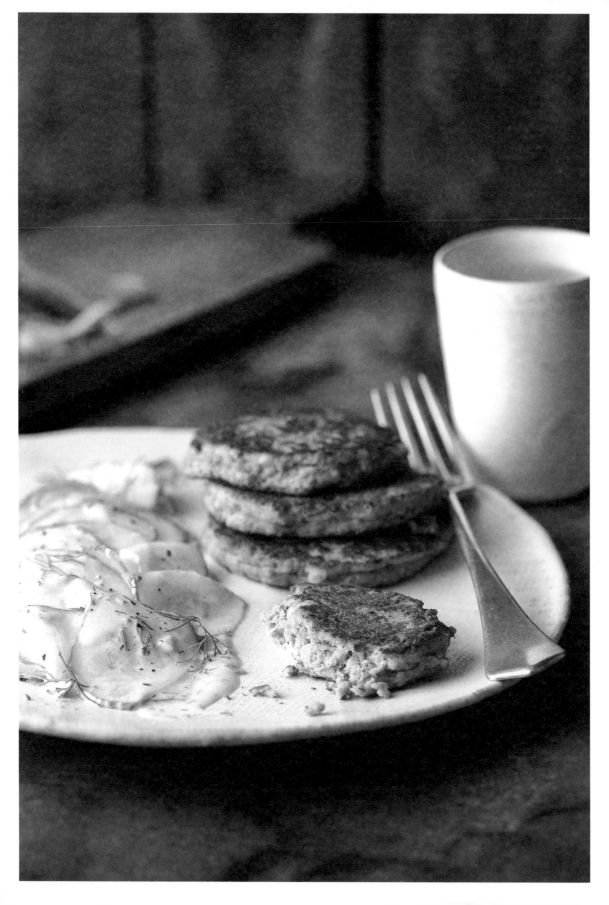

TUNA FISHCAKES WITH CUCUMBER SALAD

FOR THE FISHCAKES

1 small carrot, peeled and chopped into roughly ¾ in (2 cm) cubes
5-oz (150-g) can tuna (drained weight)
2 tablespoons mayonnaise
2 medium eggs
1 tablespoon lemon juice
1 tablespoon ground psyllium husks
¼ bunch dill, finely chopped
3 teaspoons coconut oil
salt and pepper

FOR THE CUCUMBER SALAD

2 tablespoons sour cream
1 tablespoon white wine vinegar
3 teaspoons olive oil
1 teaspoon medium-hot mustard
1 cucumber, peeled and thinly sliced
salt and pepper

Serves 2
Preparation: approx. 25 minutes
Per piece: approx. 505 kcal, 27 g protein, 39 g fat, 8 g carbohydrate

Blitz the carrot, tuna, mayonnaise, eggs, lemon juice, and ground psyllium husks in a food processor until finely chopped.

Fold in half the dill, reserving the rest for the cucumber salad. Season the fishcake mixture to taste with salt and pepper and let sit for a while.

In the meantime, prepare the cucumber salad. Stir together the sour cream, white wine vinegar, olive oil, and mustard. Season to taste with salt and pepper. Stir in the reserved dill. Combine all the ingredients with the sliced cucumber in a bowl and set aside.

Heat the coconut oil in a non-stick pan over medium heat. Using moist hands, shape four flat fishcakes from the mixture and fry them for 3–4 minutes on each side. The fishcakes are fragile so use two spatulas to help you turn them.

Divide the cucumber salad between two plates, arrange the tuna fishcakes on top, and serve.

FOR YOUR FREEZER

These tuna fishcakes can be frozen in batches for the perfect instant meal. Just let them defrost overnight in the refrigerator, then heat them up in the oven or microwave.

MARINATED TRAY-ROASTED SUMMER VEGETABLES WITH MEATBALLS

FOR THE MARINADE
juice of ½ lemon
4½ tablespoons olive oil
1 teaspoon dried basil
1 teaspoon dried oregano
salt and pepper

FOR THE VEGETABLES
1 fennel bulb, halved, stalk removed and
    thinly sliced
1 zucchini, halved and cut diagonally
    into ¼ in (5 mm) slices
1¾ oz (50 g) green beans, halved
3½ oz (100 g) cherry tomatoes

FOR THE MEATBALLS
1 small onion, finely diced
¾ oz (20 g) Gouda, roughly grated
5 oz (150 g) mixed ground beef, pork,
    or lamb
1 teaspoon mustard
freshly grated nutmeg
salt and pepper

Serves 2
Preparation: approx. 20 minutes
Cooking: approx. 20 minutes
Per portion: approx. 480 kcal, 22 g
protein, 40 g fat, 8 g carbohydrate

Preheat the oven to 400°F (200°C). Line a baking tray with parchment paper.

To make the marinade, stir the lemon juice into the olive oil, basil, and oregano. Season generously to taste with salt and pepper.

Spread all the vegetables over the baking tray, mixing them together as you do so. Drizzle evenly with the marinade.

Work the onion and Gouda into the ground meat along with the mustard and nutmeg. Season to taste with salt and pepper. Use your hands to shape eight meatballs from the mixture, then place them on top of the vegetables, and slide the tray into the center of the oven. Bake for about 20 minutes, remove from the oven, and divide between two plates to serve.

VARY YOUR VEG

There are virtually no constraints when it comes to selecting the vegetables. You can choose whatever happens to be on special offer, is in season, needs using up from your refrigerator, or appeals to your particular tastes. It might be cauliflower, eggplant, broccoli, or celery—anything goes.

CHEESE TORTILLAS
WITH GUACAMOLE

FOR THE TORTILLAS

¾ oz (50 g) Parmesan, finely grated

2 medium eggs

⅓ cup (100 g) sour cream

¼ cup (50 ml) milk

pinch of salt

2 tablespoons ground psyllium husks

2 tablespoons sesame seed flour

2 tablespoons almond flour

1 teaspoon baking powder

FOR THE FILLING

3 teaspoons coconut oil

5 oz (150 g) ground beef

1 tablespoon tomato purée

½ teaspoon ground coriander

½ teaspoon dried oregano

3½ oz (100 g) iceberg lettuce, sliced into
     thin strips

salt and pepper

FOR THE GUACAMOLE

juice of ¼ lemon

flesh of ¼ avocado

1 tablespoon crème fraîche

salt and pepper

Serves 2

Preparation: approx. 30 minutes

Per portion: approx. 775 kcal, 48 g
protein, 59 g fat, 10 g carbohydrate

Preheat the oven to 400°F (200°C). Line a baking tray with parchment paper.

Stir the Parmesan together with the eggs, sour cream, milk, salt, and ¼ cup (50 ml) of water in a bowl. In a second bowl, combine the ground psyllium husks, sesame seed flour, almond flour, and baking powder, then swiftly stir these dry ingredients into the wet ingredients.

Divide the mixture into four and shape into balls. Arrange these on the baking tray and use damp hands to press each one flat to create a roughly ¼-in (6-mm) thick tortilla. Put the tray in the center of the oven and bake for 10 minutes. Switch off the oven, open the door slightly, and leave the tortillas inside to stay warm.

In the meantime, put the coconut oil in a pan over medium heat and sauté the ground beef for about 8 minutes until crumbly and brown. Stir in the tomato purée and 1 tablespoon of water, add the coriander and oregano, and season with salt and pepper.

Add the lemon juice to a blender with the avocado and crème fraîche, and process until you have a purée. Season to taste with salt and pepper.

Remove the tortillas from the oven and spread evenly with the guacamole. Use a tablespoon to scoop the ground beef onto one half of each tortilla, and then scatter the iceberg lettuce on top. Fold up the tortillas and arrange on two plates to serve.

GUACAMOLE VARIATIONS

Have you got some leftover broccoli or asparagus from a previous day? You can use these vegetables instead of avocado to make the guacamole. Just replace the avocado with 1¾ oz (50 g) cooked vegetables and create any number of fantastic alternative options.

SOUVLAKI KEBABS
WITH MARINATED FETA

FOR THE FETA

3½ oz (100 g) feta, cut into ¾ in
    (2 cm) cubes
½ red onion, thinly sliced
1 garlic clove, roughly sliced
1 mild red chili, sliced into thin rings
1 teaspoon dried thyme
3 teaspoons olive oil
salt

FOR THE SOUVLAKI

1 tablespoon lemon juice
2 tablespoons olive oil
3 sprigs parsley, finely chopped
½ teaspoon dried rosemary
1 teaspoon dried oregano
5 oz (150 g) pork neck, chopped into
    roughly 1¼ in (3 cm) cubes
2 yellow bell peppers, chopped into
    roughly 1¼ in (3 cm) pieces
salt and pepper

Serves 2
Preparation: approx. 30 minutes
Marinating: approx. 1 hour
Per portion: approx. 495 kcal, 23 g
protein, 42 g fat, 5 g carbohydrate

Add all the feta ingredients to a bowl with a pinch of salt and carefully combine by hand so that the feta is nicely covered with the oil. Cover and chill in the refrigerator until you are ready to serve.

Mix the lemon juice with 1 tablespoon of the olive oil and the herbs in a large bowl. Season generously to taste with salt and pepper. Coat the meat with the herby marinade. Cover and chill in the refrigerator for 1 hour or overnight.

Meanwhile, soak two 8 in (20 cm) skewers in water for about 1 hour. Remove the meat from its marinade and alternately slide the chunks onto the skewers with two or three pieces of pepper in between.

Heat the remaining olive oil in a grill pan or frying pan over medium heat. Fry the souvlaki skewers for 2–3 minutes on all sides. Any pepper pieces that didn't fit on the skewers can be fried at the same time.

Remove the garlic from the feta marinade and discard. Serve the cubed feta and marinade on two plates, arrange the souvlaki skewers on top, and you are ready to eat.

LESS HEAT?

From a mild kick to infernal heat, chilies vary hugely in terms of their power. Depending on the particular variety; you may want to remove the chili seeds and white membrane to make the heat a bit milder.

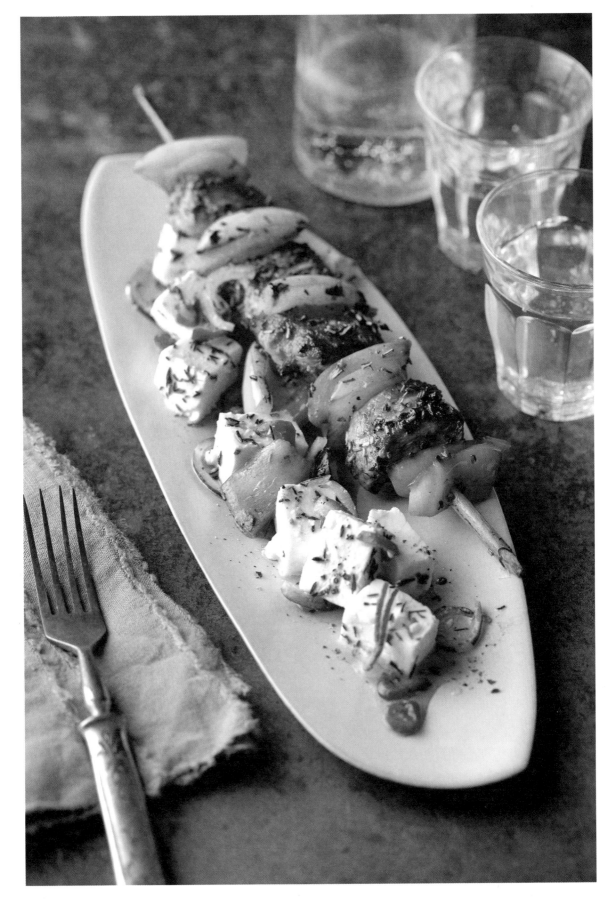

MOUSSAKA

2 eggplants, sliced lengthwise into
   $^{1}/_{3}$-in (8-mm) thick slices
1 tablespoon lemon juice
3 tablespoons olive oil
3½ oz (100 g) ground beef
1 onion, finely chopped
½ teaspoon fennel seeds
7 oz (200 g) chopped tomatoes (canned)
2½ tablespoons vegetable stock
2 bay leaves
1 teaspoon dried oregano
¾ oz (50 g) Gouda, roughly grated
1 medium egg
¼ cup (50 g) cream
freshly grated nutmeg
salt and pepper

Serves 2
Preparation: approx. 25 minutes
Cooking: approx. 45 minutes
Per portion: approx. 475 kcal, 25 g
protein, 38 g fat, 9 g carbohydrate

Preheat the oven to 425°F (220°C).

Line a baking sheet with parchment paper and place the eggplant slices flat on the sheet. Mix the lemon juice with 1 tablespoon of the olive oil and brush evenly over the eggplant. Season the slices with a pinch of salt and pepper, slide the tray into the center of the oven, and bake for 15 minutes. Remove, then reduce the oven temperature to 350°F (180°C).

In the meantime, heat the remaining olive oil in a pan and fry the ground beef until brown and crumbly. Add the onion and fennel seeds. Pour over the tomatoes and stock and add the bay leaves and oregano. Simmer everything, uncovered, for 5 minutes, then season to taste with salt and pepper. Remove the bay leaves.

Mix the Gouda into the egg and cream. Season with a pinch salt and some nutmeg.

Line the base of a 10 × 8 in (26 × 20 cm) baking dish with a third of the baked eggplant slices. Spread half the ground meat mixture on top. Cover with another layer of eggplant, spread the remaining ground meat on top, and finish with a layer of the remaining eggplant.

Pour the egg and cream sauce over the top. Transfer the baking dish to the center of the oven and bake the moussaka for 30 minutes. Remove from the oven and serve on two plates.

ZUCCHINI MOUSSAKA

You could also use 2 large zucchini instead of the eggplants. Follow the recipe as given, but only prebake the zucchini for 10 minutes, as it cooks rather more quickly than eggplant.

OVEN-ROASTED ZUCCHINI

(V)

2 zucchini, quartered lengthwise then
    cut into 3–4 pieces
zest of ½ lemon
1 garlic clove, finely chopped or crushed
4½ tablespoons olive oil
½ teaspoon nigella seeds
2 tablespoons sesame seeds
2 oz (60 g) Parmesan, finely grated
salt and pepper

Serves 2
Preparation: approx. 15 minutes
Cooking: approx. 20 minutes
Per portion: approx. 430 kcal, 16 g
protein, 38 g fat, 5 g carbohydrate

Preheat the oven to 400°F (200°C). Line a baking tray with
parchment paper.

Put the zucchini pieces into a bowl with the lemon zest, garlic,
and olive oil and toss everything by hand until the pieces are
completely coated.

Spread the zucchini evenly over the baking tray, season with
salt and pepper, and scatter over the nigella and sesame
seeds. Transfer the tray to the center of the oven and cook for
10 minutes.

Remove, sprinkle over the Parmesan, then continue baking the
zucchini for a further 8 minutes. Divide the roasted zucchini
between two plates to serve.

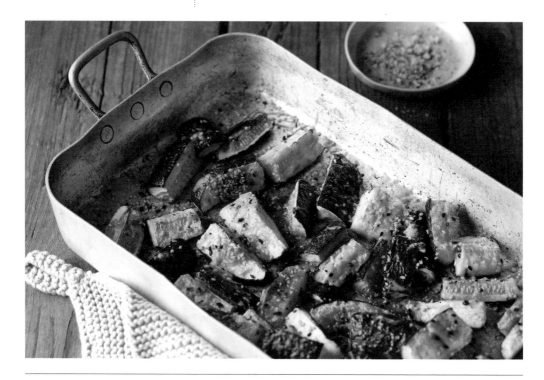

SWISS CHARD WRAPS
WITH A HAM FILLING

8 Swiss chard leaves, leaves and stalks
    separated, stalks cubed
8 slices cooked ham
4 slices Gouda, halved
8 teaspoons butter
scant ½ cup (100 ml) vegetable stock
¼ cup (50 g) cream
1 tablespoon herb cream cheese
1 teaspoon ground turmeric
salt and pepper

Serves 2
Preparation: approx. 25 minutes
Per portion: approx. 515 kcal,
37 g protein, 39 g fat, 2 g carbohydrate

Spread the Swiss chard leaves out flat on the work surface and top with the ham. Lay the Gouda slices lengthwise toward the center of the slices of ham. Fold in the sides of the Swiss chard leaves toward the center, then roll each one up and secure with a toothpick.

Add the butter to a shallow pan over medium heat and sauté the Swiss chard stalks for 2 minutes. Pour in the vegetable stock and cream, stir in the herb cream cheese, and add the turmeric. Bring to a boil, then add the Swiss chard parcels.

Simmer the parcels, covered, for about 12 minutes over low heat. Season the Swiss chard and cream cheese mixture with salt and pepper and then serve on two plates.

STUFFED EGGPLANT AU GRATIN

FOR THE EGGPLANT

3 teaspoons olive oil

1 eggplant, sliced lengthwise into
    6–8 ½-in (1 cm) thick slices

1 small red onion, finely diced

5 oz (150 g) mixed ground beef, pork,
    or lamb

1 medium egg

1 teaspoon mild paprika

salt and pepper

FOR THE BÉCHAMEL SAUCE

4 teaspoons butter

1 teaspoon ground psyllium husks

pinch of ground cloves

freshly grated nutmeg

¼ cup (50 ml) milk

1½ oz (40 g) cheddar, roughly grated

salt and pepper

Serves 2

Preparation: approx. 30 minutes

Cooking: approx. 30 minutes

Per portion: approx. 500 kcal, 25 g
protein, 42 g fat, 5 g carbohydrate

Heat the olive oil in a large non-stick pan. Sauté the sliced eggplant in the oil for 1 minute on each side, remove, and drain on some paper towel.

Put the onion, ground meat, and egg into a bowl and work together by hand. Add the paprika and season with salt and pepper.

Place the eggplant slices side by side on a work surface. Put 1 tablespoon of the ground meat mixture onto half of each eggplant slice (on the side with the largest surface area) and fold the other half over the top. Press down slightly to distribute the meat mixture. Transfer these eggplant pockets to a 10 × 8 in (26 × 20 cm) baking dish. Preheat the oven to 350°F (180°C).

Melt the butter in a pan. Using a whisk, stir the ground psyllium husks into the melted butter. Add the ground cloves, season with nutmeg, salt, and pepper, then add ⅔ cup (150 ml) of water and the milk while stirring constantly. Bring to a boil over medium heat until the sauce has thickened. This will take 2–4 minutes.

Remove the pan from the heat, stir in the cheddar, and pour the sauce evenly over the eggplant parcels. Bake the dish in the center of the oven for 25–30 minutes until the béchamel sauce is golden brown. Remove from the oven and divide between two plates to serve.

STUFFED BELL PEPPERS

You can also use this filling for stuffed bell peppers. To do this, slice 1 yellow bell pepper in half and remove the seeds and membrane. Scoop the ground meat mixture into the pepper halves, then transfer them to an 8-in (20-cm) square, lightly greased baking dish. Pour over the béchamel sauce and bake as described.

ZUCCHINI OMELET
WITH SERRANO HAM

4 medium eggs
4 teaspoons cream
1 oz (30 g) pecorino, roughly grated
1 zucchini, roughly grated
1 garlic clove, finely chopped or crushed
6 pitted black olives, chopped
1 teaspoon mild paprika
3 tablespoons olive oil
1 tomato, finely diced
3 slices serrano ham
salt and pepper

Serves 2
Preparation: approx. 20 minutes
Per portion: approx. 470 kcal, 21 g
protein, 42 g fat, 4 g carbohydrate

Whisk the eggs in a bowl with the cream. Add the cheese, zucchini, tomatoes garlic, olives, and paprika and stir well. Season with a pinch of salt and pepper.

Heat 1 tablespoon of the oil in a non-stick pan. Add the egg mixture, cover, and cook over medium heat for 8 minutes. Slip the omelet onto a plate. Place a second plate upside down over the top, then flip both plates over together to turn the omelet.

Add the remaining oil to the pan. Slide the omelet back into the pan from the second plate, cover, and continue cooking for 5 minutes.

Slip the omelet onto a chopping board, slice into quarters, top with the ham, and serve.

ALTERNATIVE FILLINGS

Omelets are great for using up any leftovers. Do you have some cooked vegetables or a bit of meat that needs finishing? Chop them into little pieces and use these instead of the zucchini or tomato in the egg mixture. This way you'll always be able to rustle up new varieties of omelet.

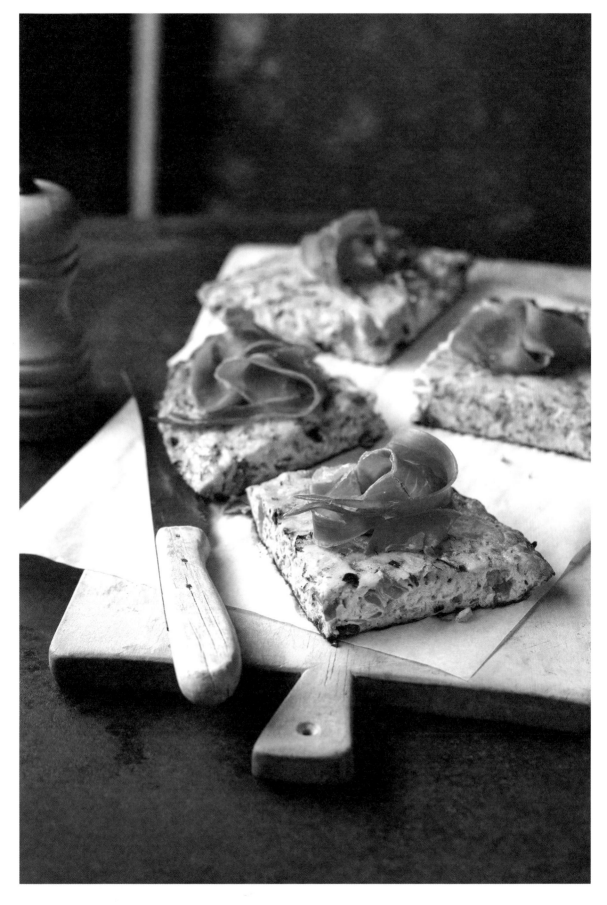

CHICKEN NUGGETS
WITH BAKED TOMATOES

2 tomatoes, halved

1½ tablespoons pine nuts, roughly
chopped

¾ oz (20 g) Parmesan, finely grated

1 scallion, sliced into very thin rings

1 tablespoon creamed coconut

2 tablespoons Greek yogurt

1 teaspoon curry powder

¼ apple, finely grated

2 tablespoons ground almonds

8 teaspoons clarified butter

4½ oz (120 g) chicken breast, cut into
roughly 1¼ in (3 cm) cubes

1 medium egg, beaten

salt and pepper

Serves 2

Preparation: approx. 35 minutes

Per portion: approx. 610 kcal,
27 g protein, 52 g fat, 8 g carbohydrate

Place the tomato halves in an 8-in (20-cm) square baking dish, cut-side up. Mix the pine nuts with the Parmesan and scallion. Season the tomatoes with salt and pepper and sprinkle with this mixture. Slide the dish into the center of a cold oven and set the temperature to 400°F (200°C) to cook for 25 minutes.

Meanwhile, stir together the creamed coconut, yogurt, and curry powder. Stir the apple into the curry sauce and season to taste with salt and pepper. Put the almonds on a flat plate.

Warm the clarified butter in a pan over medium heat. Season the chicken pieces with salt and pepper and toss them in the egg, then in the almonds. Fry the pieces for 2 minutes on each side until golden brown all over. Remove from the pan, drain on paper towel, and serve on two plates. Take the tomatoes out of the oven, arrange on the plates, and serve with the curry sauce.

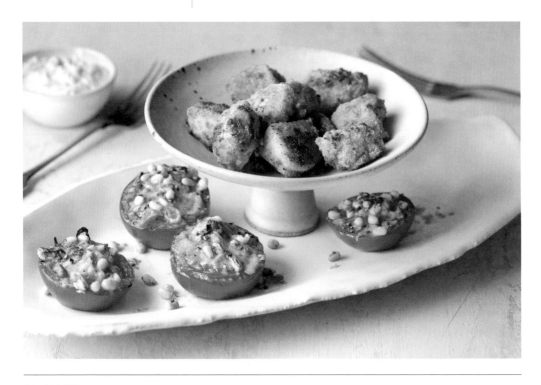

CAULIFLOWER AND TURMERIC CHEESE FRITTERS

(V)

3¼ cups (400 g) cauliflower florets
3½ oz (100 g) Gouda, roughly grated
2 medium eggs
¼ cup (50 g) full-fat cream cheese
freshly grated nutmeg
1 teaspoon ground turmeric
2 teaspoons ground psyllium husks
3 tablespoons coconut oil
salt and pepper

Serves 2
Preparation: approx. 25 minutes
Per portion: approx. 465 kcal,
29 g protein, 36 g fat, 8 g carbohydrate

Bring about 2 cups (500 ml) of water to a boil and add salt. Cook the cauliflower florets in the boiling water for 6 minutes, covered, then drain. Immerse in cold water to prevent them cooking any further, then drain again.

Meanwhile, mix the Gouda with the eggs and cream cheese. Blitz the cauliflower in a food processor until you have fine crumbs, then add it to the egg and cheese mixture. Season with salt, pepper, and nutmeg, then add the turmeric and ground psyllium husks and stir briskly. Let sit for roughly 10 minutes.

Add the oil to a non-stick pan over medium heat. Use damp hands to shape eight fritters from the mix, and then fry for 4 minutes on each side. Remove and drain on some paper towel before serving.

SERVE WITH A SIDE

Mix a handful each of iceberg lettuce and radicchio cut into strips. Make a dressing by stirring together ½ teaspoon medium-hot mustard, 2 tablespoons red wine vinegar, and 1 tablespoon olive oil and season generously with salt and pepper. Toss the salad in the dressing.

TOMATO AND RED BELL PEPPER
SOUP WITH PARMESAN CHIPS

(V)

FOR THE PARMESAN CHIPS

1 teaspoon chili flakes

1 tablespoon fennel seeds

2 oz (60 g) Parmesan, finely grated

FOR THE SOUP

1 red bell pepper, halved and deseeded

3 tablespoons olive oil

1 small onion, finely chopped

7 oz (200 g) peeled tomatoes (canned)

1 cup (250 ml) vegetable stock

1 teaspoon dried rosemary

2 sprigs basil, leaves picked

2 tablespoons crème fraîche

salt and pepper

Serves 2

Preparation: approx. 30 minutes

Per portion: approx. 395 kcal, 15 g
protein, 32 g fat, 10 g carbohydrate

Preheat the oven to 400°F (200°C). Line a baking tray with parchment paper. Crush the chili flakes and fennel seeds using a pestle and mortar and mix with the Parmesan.

Dollop spoonfuls of the mixture on the baking tray to create six Parmesan chips. Space them somewhat apart because they will spread. Slide the tray into the center of the oven and bake for 4 minutes until the cheese has melted and the edges have begun to go brown. Remove from the oven and let cool completely on a wire rack (still on the parchment paper). Set the oven to the broiler setting.

To make the soup, place the pepper pieces skin-side up on a baking tray and bake on the top shelf of the oven for 10–15 minutes until the skin begins to blister and turn black. Remove, cover with a clean, wet dish towel, and let cool slightly.

Meanwhile, add the olive oil to a pan over medium heat and sweat the onion for 2 minutes. Add the peeled tomatoes to the pan along with the vegetable stock, rosemary, and basil and bring to a boil uncovered. Simmer for 8–10 minutes.

Pull the skin off the pepper and add the peeled pieces to the pan. Blend with a hand blender, return to a boil, and season to taste with salt and pepper.

Serve in two deep bowls, each one topped with 1 tablespoon crème fraîche and garnished with the Parmesan chips.

SPEED THINGS UP

This soup still tastes great without the time-consuming step of roasting the peppers to remove the skin. Once blended the skin is barely noticeable.

VEGGIE SPAGHETTI
WITH MUSHROOM SAUCE

(V)

FOR THE VEGGIE SPAGHETTI
1 kohlrabi, peeled and spiralized
1 large carrot, peeled and spiralized
1 small zucchini, spiralized
3 sprigs parsley, roughly chopped
salt

FOR THE MUSHROOM SAUCE
8 teaspoons butter
1 small onion, finely diced
7 oz (200 g) button mushrooms, halved
    or quartered
2/3 cup (150 g) cream
1/4 cup (50 g) full-fat cream cheese
1/2 teaspoon mild paprika
freshly grated nutmeg
salt and pepper

Serves 2
Preparation: approx. 25 minutes
Per portion: approx. 520 kcal, 10 g
protein, 48 g fat, 12 g carbohydrate

Bring approx. 6 cups (1.5 liters) salted water to a boil in a pan. Boil the veggie noodles, uncovered, for 4 minutes, then drain.

Meanwhile, add the butter to a pan over high heat. Sauté the onion and mushrooms together for 2 minutes.

Pour in the cream, bring to a boil, uncovered, and allow to thicken slightly for 1 minute. Remove the pan from the heat and stir in the cream cheese. Add the paprika and season the mushrooms to taste with nutmeg, salt, and pepper. Cover to keep warm.

Divide the veggie noodles between two deep plates. Pour over the mushroom sauce and scatter with chopped parsley to serve.

DELICIOUS RECYCLING
When preparing broccoli, the stalk often ends up unused in the compost, but it's ideal for making veggie spaghetti. Just peel it, then use it in exactly the same way as you would a carrot. Depending on the time of year, you can also make wonderful veggie spaghetti from sweet potato (in moderation), beets, and pumpkin. If you don't have a spiralizer, you can use a peeler to make thin strips like tagliatelle.

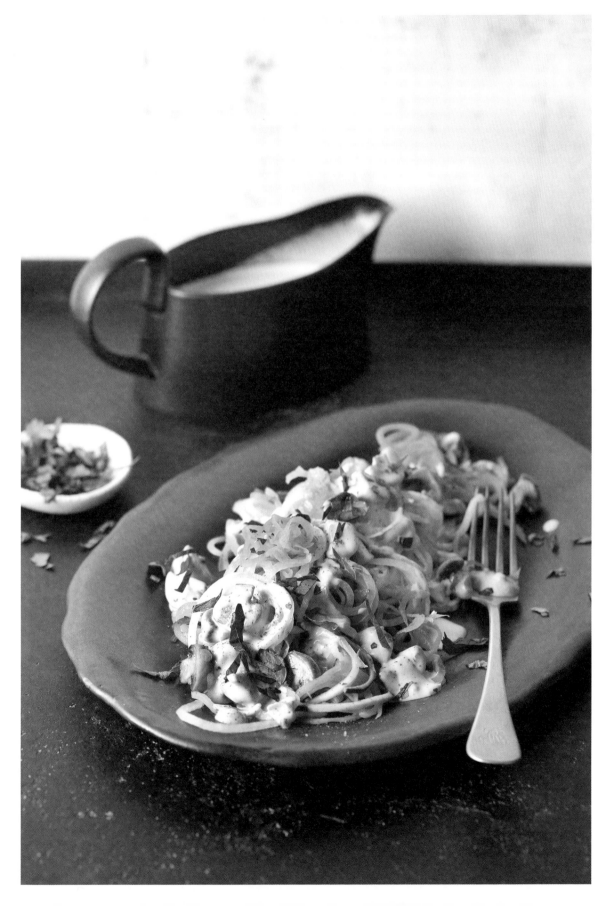

SAUERKRAUT AND BACON PATTIES

10½ oz (300 g) sauerkraut
4 strips bacon, finely diced
1 carrot, peeled and roughly grated
1¾ oz (50 g) celery root, peeled and
    roughly grated
½ red bell pepper, cut into thin strips
2 tablespoons ground psyllium husks
2 medium eggs
½ teaspoon nigella seeds
½ cup (150 g) Greek yogurt
1 tablespoon ajvar
3 tablespoons coconut oil
salt and pepper

Serves 2
Preparation: approx. 25 minutes
Per portion: approx. 340 kcal,
9 g protein, 29 g fat, 10 g carbohydrate

Fork through the sauerkraut and add the bacon and vegetables. Likewise, add the ground psyllium husks, eggs, nigella seeds, and a pinch each of salt and pepper. Combine the mixture with your hands and let sit for 10 minutes.

Stir together the yogurt and ajvar and season to taste with salt and pepper. Put the coconut oil in a non-stick pan over low heat. With damp hands, shape six flat patties from the mixture and then fry them in the covered pan for 5–6 minutes on each side. Arrange the patties on two plates and serve with the dip.

PUMPKIN AND SAUERKRAUT PATTIES
Replace the carrot, celery root, and pepper with 7 oz (200 g) pumpkin (Hokkaido or butternut squash). Roughly grate the pumpkin or squash, then proceed as described above.

CAULIFLOWER AND SPINACH BAKE

1 small cauliflower, split into florets
8 teaspoons butter
1 small onion, finely diced
7 oz (200 g) spinach
¼ cup (50 g) cream
4½ oz (125 g) ball mozzarella, diced or
    grated
1¾ oz (50 g) Gouda, roughly grated
pinch of ground cloves
freshly grated nutmeg
salt and pepper

Serves 2
Preparation: approx. 25 minutes
Cooking: approx. 20 minutes
Per portion: approx. 495 kcal, 25 g
protein, 41 g fat, 6 g carbohydrate

In a medium-sized pan, bring roughly 6 cups (1.5 liters) water to a boil and add salt. Boil the cauliflower florets for 8 minutes until just done, then briefly drain.

Meanwhile, heat 4 teaspoons of the butter in a shallow pan. Sauté the onion for 1 minute, then add the spinach and let it wilt before setting the pan aside. Preheat the oven to 400°F (200°C).

Blitz the cauliflower in a food-processor with the cream and the remaining butter until crumbly. Mix with the spinach, mozzarella, and Gouda. Add the cloves and season with nutmeg, salt, and pepper. Transfer to an 8-in (20-cm) square baking dish and cook in the center of the oven for 20 minutes until the cheese is golden brown. Remove from the dish and serve on two plates.

BRAISED PORK TENDERLOIN
WITH PAPRIKA MUSHROOMS

7 oz (200 g) pork tenderloin, sliced into
    roughly 1½ in (4 cm) cubes
3 tablespoons coconut oil
1 small onion, thinly sliced
1 tablespoon tomato purée
1¾ cups (400 ml) meat stock
4 teaspoons butter
14 oz (400 g) button mushrooms,
    quartered
scant ½ cup (100 g) cream
½ teaspoon dried thyme
1 teaspoon mild paprika
freshly grated nutmeg
salt and pepper

Serves 2
Preparation: approx. 45 minutes
Per portion: approx. 515 kcal, 29 g
protein, 43 g fat, 5 g carbohydrate

Generously season the pork tenderloin with salt and pepper. Put the coconut oil in a pan over medium heat and sauté the meat on all sides for 5 minutes until golden brown.

Add the onion to the pan and continue frying for 10 minutes. Once the meat and onion have acquired plenty of color, stir in the tomato purée and cook for a further 1 minute.

Pour over the stock and cover the pan with a lid. Braise for 30 minutes over medium heat. Check occasionally to make sure there is enough liquid in the pan, and top up with hot water if necessary.

Meanwhile, melt the butter in a pan over medium heat and sauté the mushrooms briskly until they begin to brown. Add the mushrooms to the meat and pour in the cream.

Bring to a boil over high heat and simmer for 4–5 minutes to reduce the sauce to a creamy consistency. Add the dried thyme and paprika and season with some nutmeg, salt, and pepper. Serve on two plates.

A TASTY ALTERNATIVE

Braising means the pork tenderloin won't get too dry. If preferred, you can use diced pork neck instead. The stewing meat will need about 20 minutes longer to cook to make sure it is nice and soft once braised. You will need to keep checking the liquid levels and topping the dish up with hot water. Most of the liquid will be cooked off subsequently when you reduce the sauce.

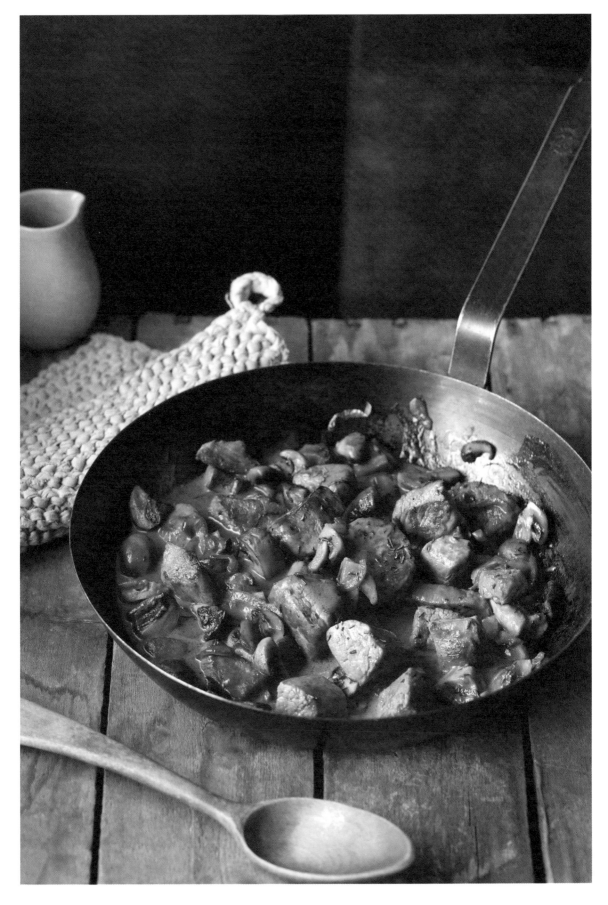

COUNTRY CASSEROLE
WITH BELL PEPPER

3 tablespoons coconut oil
7 oz (200 g) ground beef
1 small red onion, finely diced
1 tablespoon tomato purée
5 oz (150 g) button mushrooms,
    quartered
1 small zucchini, cubed
1 yellow bell pepper, diced into ¾ in (2
    cm) cubes
1 mild red chili, sliced into thin rings
scant 2 cups (450 ml) vegetable stock
2 bay leaves
1 teaspoon dried thyme
2 tablespoons full-fat cream cheese
salt and pepper

Serves 2
Preparation: approx. 25 minutes
Per portion: approx. 450 kcal, 26 g
protein, 35 g fat, 7 g carbohydrate

Put the oil in a pan over medium heat. Fry the ground beef until browned, stirring frequently. Add the onion to the pan and continue cooking.

Stir the tomato purée into the ground beef and cook for a further 1 minute. Add the vegetables and chili and pour over the vegetable stock. Add the bay leaves and thyme and bring to a boil. Reduce to medium heat and simmer, uncovered, for 8–10 minutes. Stir in the cream cheese, season with salt and pepper, and serve immediately.

A HINT OF SPICE
Prepare this dish with ground lamb and flavor with ½ teaspoon each of ground cumin and coriander, 1 teaspoon ras el hanout (or other chilli mix), and 6 mint leaves cut into strips.

ZUCCHINI AND MOZZARELLA BOATS WITH A HERB SAUCE

2 small zucchini, halved lengthwise
4½ oz (120 g) mixed ground beef, pork, or lamb
4½ oz (125 g) ball mozzarella, finely diced
1 teaspoon dried rosemary
4 strips bacon
¼ cup (50 g) cream
2 tablespoons herb cream cheese
salt and pepper

Serves 2
Preparation: approx. 20 minutes
Cooking: approx. 25 minutes
Per portion: approx. 525 kcal, 31 g protein, 42 g fat, 5 g carbohydrate

Preheat the oven to 400°F (200°C). Use a spoon to hollow out the zucchini slightly, then chop up the scooped-out flesh and add it to a bowl with the ground meat.

Add the mozzarella to the ground meat and work everything together using your hands until well combined. Add rosemary, salt, and pepper and transfer into the zucchini halves. Top each zucchini boat with a strip of bacon. Transfer them to a 10 × 8 in (26 × 20 cm) baking dish and then into the center of the oven and bake for 15 minutes.

Stir together the cream, herb cream cheese, and 1 tablespoon of water until smooth. Briefly take the dish out of the oven, pour the herby cream sauce over the zucchini, and return the dish to the oven. Cook for a further 10 minutes. Remove, and serve the zucchini on two plates.

BEEF SOUP

9 oz (250 g) beef for stewing (shank or
  brisket)
bunch of soup vegetables (carrot, celery
  root, leek)
1 onion
1 garlic clove
4 juniper berries
½ teaspoon dried thyme
½ teaspoon black peppercorns
8 teaspoons butter
3 sprigs parsley, finely chopped
salt

Serves 2
Preparation: approx. 20 minutes
Cooking: approx. 2 hours
Per portion: approx. 510 kcal, 24 g
protein, 44 g fat, 5 g carbohydrate

Add the stewing meat to a pan and cover with 6 cups (1.5 liters) cold water. Bring to a boil, uncovered, over medium heat, then lower the temperature so that it just simmers gently.

Meanwhile, prepare the soup vegetables. Wash and peel the carrot and celery root, carefully clean the leek. Add any peelings into the pan with the meat. Set aside the soup vegetables.

Halve the unpeeled onion, fry it in a non-stick pan with no oil, cut-surface facing down until it is almost black, then add it with skin still on to the meat pan. Crush the unpeeled garlic clove and add this to the pan. Grind the juniper berries using a pestle and mortar and add these to the pan along with the thyme and peppercorns.

Simmer the broth, uncovered, for 2 hours. If necessary, lower the temperature to prevent it boiling too vigorously. If any foam appears on the surface you should scoop this off using a slotted spoon. After the 2 hours, remove the meat from the stock and let cool slightly.

Meanwhile, chop the prepared soup vegetables into roughly ½ in (1 cm) cubes. Heat the butter in a large pan and sauté the chopped vegetables for 5 minutes. Pour the stock through a fine sieve directly onto the vegetables in the pan and bring to a boil. Simmer for 10 minutes.

Meanwhile, chop the meat into ½ in (1 cm) cubes and add these to the soup. Season the soup with salt, scatter over the parsley, and serve in two soup bowls.

STOCK ON SUPPLY

Making a rich stock using beef involves a bit of work and takes some time—but it's well worth the effort for the flavor. To make it even more worthwhile, why not prepare four times the quantity of stock then decant it into three or four sterile jam jars while still boiling hot. If stored in the refrigerator, these will keep for up to 3 months.

4

DINNER

Whether slow bakes or fast schnitzel, dinner needs to be something worth coming home for. Think ahead and be sure you have everything organized before you get started in the kitchen. Take your time. Good things are worth waiting for.

PORK MEDALLIONS WITH
A TOMATO AND PEPPER MEDLEY

FOR THE BASIL BUTTER
2½ oz (70 g) soft butter
zest of ¼ lemon
6 basil leaves, sliced into thin strips
salt and pepper

FOR THE MEDALLIONS
AND VEGETABLES
3 teaspoons coconut oil
7 oz (200 g) pork tenderloin, sliced into
    4 medallions
3 teaspoons olive oil
1 red onion, thinly sliced
2 yellow bell peppers, diced into
    ¾ in (2 cm) cubes
3½ oz (100 g) cherry tomatoes, halved
4 sage leaves, sliced into thin strips
1 garlic clove, finely chopped or crushed
salt and pepper

Serves 2
Preparation: approx. 25 minutes
Per portion: approx. 550 kcal, 25 g
protein, 47 g fat, 8 g carbohydrate

To make the basil butter, beat the butter in a bowl until smooth. Stir in the lemon zest and the strips of basil. Season to taste with salt and pepper and chill until ready to serve.

Heat the coconut oil in a heavy-based pan. Season the medallions with salt and pepper and fry them on each side for 3–4 minutes.

Meanwhile, heat the olive oil in another pan and sauté the onion for 1 minute. Add the peppers and continue cooking for 2 minutes. Add the cherry tomatoes, sage, and garlic, season generously with salt and pepper and mix well. Cook for another 2 minutes. Put two pork medallions on each plate and serve with the vegetables and basil butter.

HERB BUTTER VARIATIONS

Other herbs in the herb butter also work well with the medallions. For instance, you could replace the basil with 1 tablespoon of chives snipped into little pieces or 2–3 wild garlic leaves cut into thin strips. You could also use the finely chopped leaves from a sprig of rosemary or the little leaves from 2–4 sprigs of thyme.

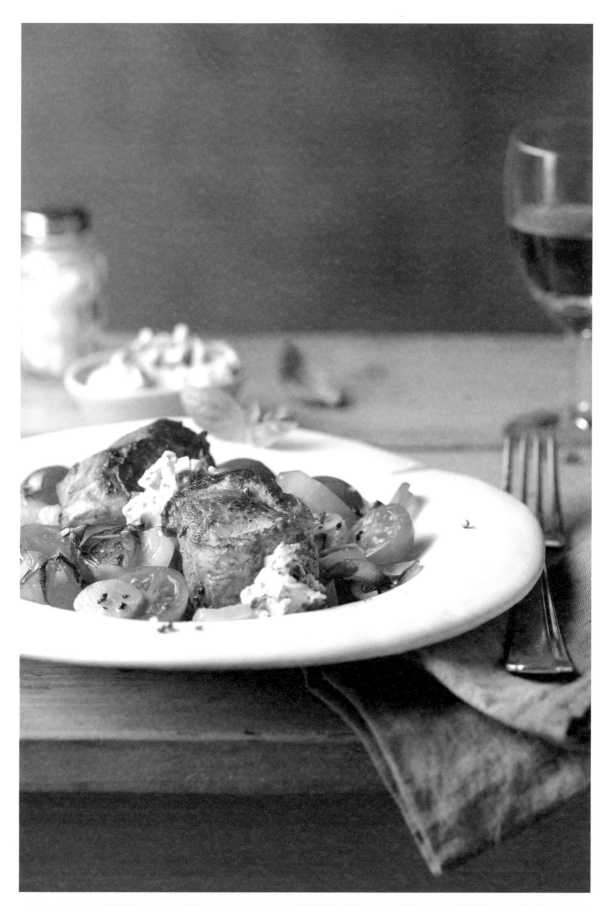

ZUCCHINI LASAGNA
WITH SOY BOLOGNESE

⅔ cup (150 ml) vegetable stock
⅓ cup/1¾ oz (50 g) fine textured
   soy protein
4½ tablespoons olive oil
2 small zucchini, sliced lengthwise into
   5 slices each
1 small onion, finely diced
5 oz (150 g) tomato puree
1 teaspoon dried basil
1 teaspoon dried thyme
salt and pepper

FOR THE BÉCHAMEL SAUCE
4 teaspoons butter
½ teaspoon ground psyllium husks
freshly grated nutmeg
pinch of ground cloves
¼ cup (50 g) cream
¾ oz (20 g) Parmesan, finely grated
salt and pepper

Serves 2
Preparation: approx. 30 minutes
Cooking: approx. 25 minutes
Per portion: approx. 510 kcal, 19 g
protein, 43 g fat, 11 g carbohydrate

Bring the vegetable stock to a boil, stir in the textured
soy protein, remove the pan from the heat and leave the soy
granules to stand for roughly 15 minutes.

Put 2 tablespoons of the olive oil in a pan over medium heat and
sauté the zucchini slices for 1 minute on each side, then remove
from the pan. Put the remaining oil in a pan over medium heat
and sauté the onion for 2 minutes until it begins to take on a bit
of color. Pour in the puree, add the soaked textured soy protein
and bring everything to a boil. Cover and simmer over low heat
for 10 minutes, add the basil and thyme, then season to taste
with salt and pepper.

Put half the sauce into an 8-in (20-cm) square baking dish and
place five slices of zucchini on top, arranging them side by side.
Cover with the remaining sauce, followed by the remaining zucchini slices. Preheat the oven to 400°F (200°C).

For the béchamel sauce, melt the butter in a shallow pan over
medium heat. Stir the ground psyllium husks into the melted
butter with a whisk. Add a pinch of nutmeg and the ground
cloves, season with salt and pepper, and pour in ¼ cup (50 ml)
water and the cream, stirring continuously. Simmer over medium
heat until the sauce thickens. Remove the pan from the heat,
stir in the Parmesan, and pour the sauce evenly over the
zucchini lasagna.

Bake in the center of the oven for 20–25 minutes until the
béchamel sauce is golden brown. Serve on two plates.

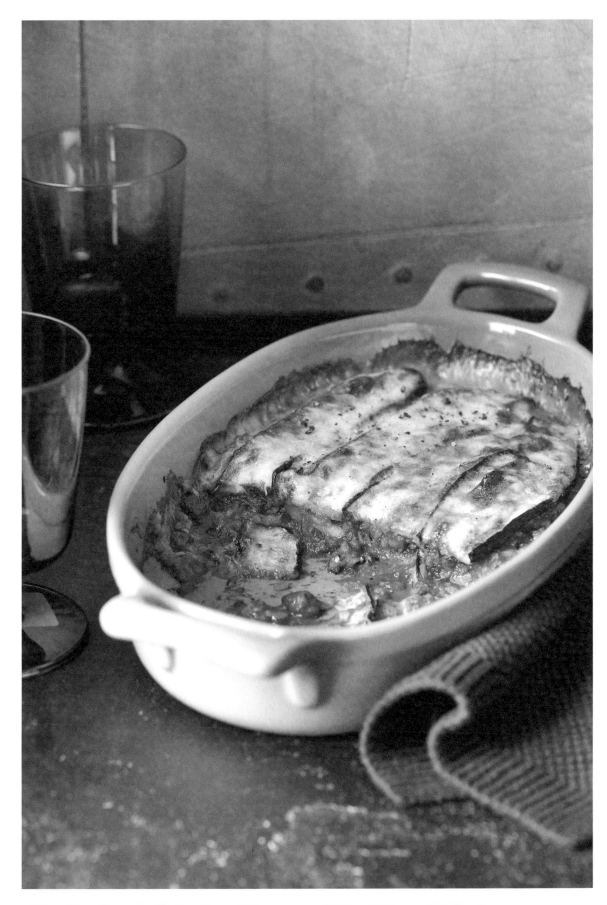

MEATBALLS WITH ASPARAGUS SALAD

3 teaspoons olive oil

14 oz (400 g) green asparagus, sliced
    into 1¼ in (3 cm) pieces

⅓ cup (80 ml) vegetable stock

¾ bunch radishes, quartered

sprig of tarragon, leaves finely chopped

1 tablespoon white wine vinegar

1 small red onion, finely chopped

1 garlic clove, finely chopped

9 oz (250 g) ground meat (beef and pork)

1 medium egg

1 tablespoon mustard

1 tablespoon coconut flour

freshly grated nutmeg

3 teaspoons coconut oil

salt and pepper

Serves 2

Preparation: approx. 30 minutes

Per portion: approx. 580 kcal, 36 g
protein, 45 g fat, 8 g carbohydrate

Put the olive oil in a large pan over medium heat. Sauté the asparagus pieces for 2 minutes, pour in the vegetable stock, and simmer over medium heat for 10 minutes.

In a bowl, toss the radishes and tarragon leaves with the asparagus and vinegar. Season to taste with salt and pepper and let sit.

In the meantime, prepare the meatballs. Add the onion and garlic to a bowl with the ground meat, egg, mustard, and coconut flour and combine. Season to taste with nutmeg, salt, and pepper.

Use your hands to form 12 equal-size balls from the mixture. Heat the coconut oil in a non-stick pan and fry the meatballs for 3–4 minutes on all sides. Divide the salad between two plates and arrange the meatballs on top to serve.

CHICKEN IN BUTTERMILK SAUCE

scant ½ cup (100 ml) buttermilk
3 tablespoons olive oil
1 teaspoon mild ground paprika
4 chicken drumsticks
8 teaspoons butter
10½ oz (300 g) white asparagus, peeled
    and woody ends trimmed
scant ½ cup (100 ml) vegetable stock
juice of ½ lemon
4 sprigs flat-leaf parsley, finely chopped,
    plus leaves to serve
salt and pepper

Serves 2
Preparation: approx. 25 minutes
Cooking: approx. 40 minutes
Per portion: approx. 465 kcal, 18 g
protein, 41 g fat, 5 g carbohydrate

Preheat the oven to 400°F (200°C). Make a marinade from the buttermilk, olive oil, and ground paprika and season generously with salt and pepper. Lay the chicken drumsticks in a 10 × 8 in (26 × 20 cm) baking dish. Pour over the marinade, put the dish in the center of the oven and bake the drumsticks for 40 minutes.

Meanwhile, melt the butter in a pan over medium heat and sauté the asparagus on all sides for a few minutes until it has begun to take on a bit of color. Pour in the vegetable stock and season with a pinch of salt. Add the lemon juice, cover, and simmer the asparagus for 15–18 minutes over low heat.

Serve the asparagus on two plates and arrange the chicken drumsticks on top. Put the buttermilk juices into a blender along with the liquid from the asparagus and process. Stir in the parsley and season to taste with salt and pepper. Garnish the chicken drumsticks and asparagus with the reserved parsley leaves and serve with the sauce.

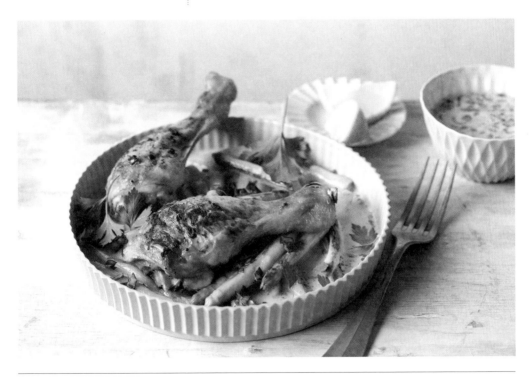

STUFFED SCHNITZEL
WITH AN ALMOND CRUST

FOR THE VEGETABLES

2 teaspoons clarified butter

1 carrot, peeled and sliced into ⅛ in
     (3 mm) discs

1 zucchini, sliced into ¼ in (5 mm) discs

⅔ cup (100 g) cherry tomatoes

¼ cup (50 ml) vegetable stock

salt and pepper

FOR THE SCHNITZEL

1 medium egg, beaten

¼ cup (25 g) ground almonds

1 pork tenderloin medallion (approx.
     5 oz/150 g), halved horizontally

1½ oz (40 g) Gorgonzola, chopped

6 teaspoons clarified butter

salt and pepper

Serves 2

Preparation: approx. 25 minutes

Per portion: approx. 505 kcal, 28 g
protein, 40 g fat, 6 g carbohydrate

To make the schnitzel, put the beaten egg into a deep dish and tip the ground almonds onto a flat plate. Place the schnitzel halves alongside each other in a freezer bag and bash them with a meat tenderizer until they are roughly ⅛ in (3 mm) thick. Scatter the Gorgonzola pieces over the schnitzels. Fold the schnitzels over and season with salt and pepper. Toss first in the beaten egg and then in the almonds.

To make the vegetables, heat the clarified butter in a pan over medium heat. First sauté the carrots for 2 minutes, then add the zucchini and cherry tomatoes, and continue cooking for a further 1 minute. Pour the stock over the vegetables and cook over medium heat for 5 minutes.

Meanwhile, to cook the schnitzel, add the clarified butter to a non-stick pan over medium heat. Fry the coated schnitzel for 4 minutes on each side. Remove the pan with the vegetables from the heat and leave it to one side until the schnitzel are ready.

Remove the schnitzel from the pan and leave to drain on some paper towel. Season the vegetables with salt and pepper and arrange on two plates. Place the schnitzel alongside the vegetables and serve.

CHOICE OF CHEESE

Of course, you can replace the Gorgonzola with any other kind of blue cheese; this only makes a very small difference in terms of the taste. If you are not so keen on the strong flavor of Gorgonzola, just substitute a milder cheese such as mozzarella, Camembert, or Gouda.

CHICKEN CURRY WITH STUFFED MUSHROOMS

FOR THE MUSHROOMS

¾ cup (100 g) frozen cauliflower florets

1 teaspoon butter, plus extra for greasing

1½ cup (160 g) brown mushrooms,
   stems removed

¼ cup (50 g) cream

freshly grated nutmeg

¾ oz (20 g) Parmesan, finely grated

salt and pepper

FOR THE CHICKEN BREAST

4 teaspoons clarified butter

5 oz (150 g) chicken breast, sliced into
   ½ in (1 cm) strips

1 small onion, finely sliced

scant ¼ cup (50 g) coconut milk (canned)

1 tablespoon creamed coconut

1 teaspoon curry powder

salt and pepper

Serves 2

Preparation: approx. 30 minutes

Per portion: approx. 455 kcal, 25 g
protein, 37 g fat, 4 g carbohydrate

In a small pan, bring 2 cups (500 ml) water to a boil and add salt. Boil the frozen cauliflower florets for 10 minutes, then drain.

Preheat the oven to 350°F (180°C). Grease the base of an 8-in (20-cm) square baking dish with butter. Place the mushrooms, open side up in the baking dish.

Put the cream and butter into the pan used to cook the cauliflower and bring to a boil, adding a pinch of freshly grated nutmeg. Add the cauliflower and process with a hand blender until it is smooth. Stir in the Parmesan and season the mix to taste with salt and pepper.

Scoop the cauliflower purée into the upturned mushrooms. Slide the dish into the center of the oven and cook the mushrooms for 15 minutes.

Add the clarified butter to a pan over medium heat. Season the chicken strips with salt and pepper and fry on all sides for 3 minutes. Add the sliced onion and continue cooking for 2 minutes. Pour in the coconut milk, then stir in the creamed coconut and curry powder. Bring to a boil and season to taste with salt and pepper.

Arrange the chicken breast with the curry sauce on two plates. Remove the mushrooms from the oven, add them to the plates and serve.

PORK CHOPS WITH AVOCADO AND APPLE SALAD

FOR THE SALAD

½ tart apple (e.g. Granny Smith), cored, quartered, and sliced into very thin slices

½ avocado, peeled, pitted, and flesh chopped into ½ in (1 cm) cubes

juice of ½ lemon

1 teaspoon mustard

3 teaspoons olive oil

½ teaspoon ground coriander

1 mild red chili, deseeded and finely chopped

¼ iceberg lettuce, sliced into roughly ½ in (1 cm) strips

salt

FOR THE PORK CHOPS

3 teaspoons coconut oil

2 pork chops (approx. 3½ oz/100 g each)

generous ¼ cup (60 g) cream

1 teaspoon green peppercorns in brine

salt and pepper

Serves 2

Preparation: approx. 20 minutes

Per portion: approx. 525 kcal, 23 g protein, 44 g fat, 5 g carbohydrate

Add the apple to a bowl with the avocado and drizzle over the lemon juice.

Put the coconut oil in a pan over high heat. Season the pork chops on both sides with salt and pepper. Fry the chops for 2 minutes on each side.

Meanwhile, make a dressing for the salad by stirring together the mustard, olive oil, coriander, and chili. Toss the avocado, apple and iceberg lettuce in the dressing. Season to taste with salt.

Remove the pork chops from the pan and wrap in aluminum foil to keep warm. Deglaze the pan with the cream, then add the green peppercorns with 1 teaspoon of the brine and simmer until the cream sauce has thickened. Season to taste with salt and pepper.

Arrange the pork chops on two plates and drizzle over the sauce. Serve the salad alongside.

LEAVE OUT THE GREEN PEPPERCORNS

Don't like green peppercorns? The sauce still tastes delicious without them. It's also particularly tasty if you add ½ teaspoon mild ground paprika or the finely chopped leaves from a sprig of rosemary.

LAMB FILLET WITH A PARSLEY AND MUSTARD TOPPING

FOR THE ZUCCHINI
AND BEAN PARCELS
4 strips bacon
1 zucchini, halved crosswise and each
    half cut lengthwise into four strips
1¾ oz (50 g) green beans, trimmed
8 teaspoons clarified butter

FOR THE LAMB FILLETS
3 sprigs of parsley, finely chopped
⅓ oz (10 g) Parmesan, finely grated
2 tablespoons ground almonds
2 lamb fillets (saddle of lamb, bone
    removed, each approx. 3½ oz/100 g)
3 teaspoons olive oil
1 teaspoon English mustard
salt and pepper

Serves 2
Preparation: approx. 25 minutes
Per portion: approx. 550 kcal, 30 g
protein, 46 g fat, 4 g carbohydrate

Preheat the oven to 400°F (200°C). Line a baking tray with parchment paper.

Spread the bacon on a work surface. Place two zucchini strips and a quarter of the beans on the end of each strip, then roll up the bacon.

Mix the parsley and Parmesan with the ground almonds.

Season the lamb fillets with salt and pepper. Add the olive oil to a pan over medium heat. Fry the lamb fillets for 2 minutes on each side. Remove from the pan and lay them on the baking tray.

Brush the top of each fillet with mustard. Spread the almond and parsley mixture evenly on top in a thick layer. Slide the tray into the center of the oven and bake the lamb fillets for 10 minutes.

Meanwhile, heat the clarified butter in the same pan in which you fried the lamb and sauté the zucchini and bean parcels for 2 minutes on each side. Add 3 tablespoons water, reduce to low heat, cover, and continue cooking for 10 minutes.

Place two zucchini bean parcels on each plate. Remove the lamb from the oven and slice each fillet twice diagonally on a chopping board to serve.

TRY RATATOUILLE WITH LAMB

Finely dice 1 small onion and sauté in 1 tablespoon of olive oil. Add 3½ oz (100 g) each of cubed eggplant, yellow pepper, and zucchini and sauté for 1 minute along with the onion. Add 7 oz (200 g) chopped tomatoes (canned), cover, and simmer over low heat for 15 minutes. Add ½ teaspoon each of dried basil and oregano and season with some salt and pepper.

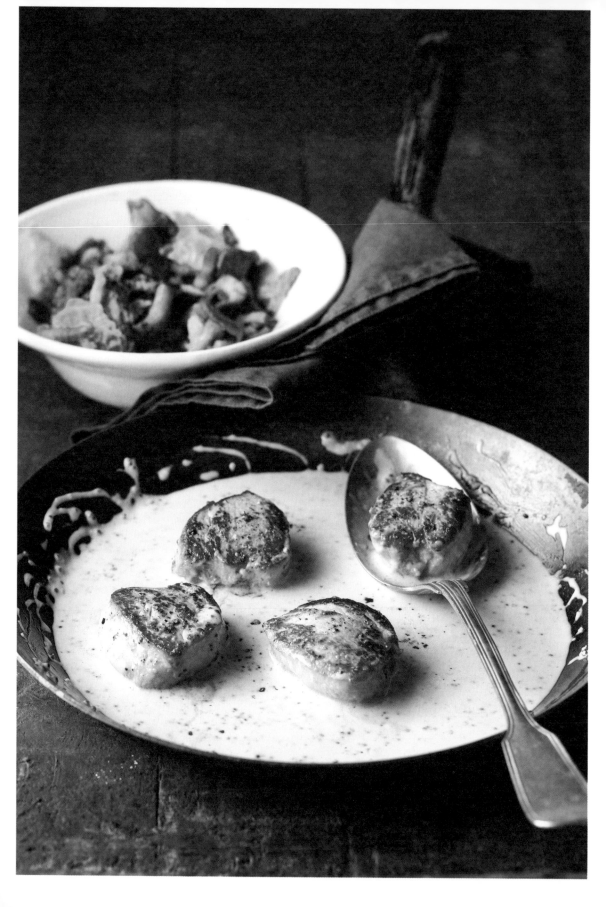

PORK TENDERLOIN IN MUSTARD SAUCE WITH SAVOY CABBAGE AND MUSHROOMS

FOR THE VEGETABLES
4 teaspoons clarified butter
7 oz (200 g) Savoy cabbage, stalk
	removed and leaves thinly sliced
5 strips bacon, diced or sliced
	into strips
3½ oz (100 g) small button mushrooms,
	or mixed wild mushrooms if you have
	them (e.g. chanterelles, bay bolete
	mushrooms, porcini), halved or
	quartered depending on size
scant ½ cup (100 ml) vegetable stock
freshly grated nutmeg
salt and pepper

FOR THE PORK TENDERLOIN
3 teaspoons coconut oil
7 oz (200 g) pork tenderloin, cut into four
	medallions
scant ½ cup (100 g) cream
1 tablespoon wholegrain Dijon mustard
salt and pepper

Serves: 2
Preparation: approx. 25 minutes
Per portion: approx. 540 kcal, 31 g
protein, 44 g fat, 5 g carbohydrate

Put the clarified butter in a pan over medium heat. Sauté the Savoy cabbage strips and bacon for 2 minutes. Add the mushrooms and continue cooking for a further 2 minutes. Pour in the vegetable stock and season with a pinch each of freshly grated nutmeg, salt, and pepper. Cover and simmer over low heat for about 15 minutes.

Add the coconut oil to a pan over medium heat. Press the pork medallions slightly flat with the palm of your hand, season with salt and pepper, and fry for 3 minutes on each side. Remove, transfer to a plate, and cover with aluminum foil to keep warm.

Deglaze the pan with the cream, stir in the mustard, and bring to a boil. Season to taste with salt and pepper. Place the medallions in the sauce and let infuse for 2 minutes.

In the meantime, season the savoy cabbage and mushroom mixture once more with salt, pepper, and nutmeg and divide between two plates. Arrange the medallions on top and serve with the sauce.

TRY WITH KALE
Try this recipe using kale, if you like it. This hearty variety of cabbage almost tastes better here and can be prepared in exactly the same way as the Savoy cabbage.

CHICKEN LEGS IN BACON SAUCE
WITH SAVOY CABBAGE

FOR THE CHICKEN LEGS
AND SAUCE
2 chicken legs
4 teaspoons coconut oil
2 strips bacon, finely chopped
1 onion, finely diced
3½ oz (100 g) mushrooms, quartered
1 teaspoon tomato purée
¼ cup (50 ml) red wine
¾ cup (200 ml) vegetable stock
½ teaspoon dried thyme
¼ cup (50 g) cream
salt and pepper

FOR THE SAVOY CABBAGE
8 teaspoons butter
7 oz (200 g) savoy cabbage, thinly sliced
freshly grated nutmeg
salt

Serves 2
Preparation: approx. 25 minutes
Cooking: approx. 40 minutes
Per portion: approx. 670 kcal, 34 g
protein, 55 g fat, 5 g carbohydrate

Season the chicken legs with salt and pepper. Add the coconut oil to a pan over medium heat and fry the chicken legs for 5 minutes until golden brown all over. Transfer them to a 10 × 8 in (26 × 20 cm) baking dish and preheat the oven to 400°F (200°C).

Fry the bacon in the hot chicken pan for 3–4 minutes, stirring occasionally. Add the onion to the bacon in the pan. Add the mushrooms to the pan and continue frying briskly for 3–5 minutes until they are golden brown.

Stir in the tomato purée followed by the red wine. Add the vegetable stock and thyme. Pour the juices over the chicken legs in the baking dish. Transfer the dish to the center of the oven and bake the chicken for 20 minutes. Turn the chicken legs and continue cooking for 20 minutes.

Heat the butter in a pan and sauté the Savoy cabbage for 2 minutes, stirring occasionally, until it has acquired a bit of color. Add 3–4 tablespoons of water, season with a generous pinch of salt and freshly grated nutmeg, cover, and cook over low heat for 15 minutes.

Remove the chicken legs from the oven, wrap in aluminum foil, and keep warm in the switched-off oven.

Transfer the bacon mixture to a pan and pour in the cream. Reduce over high heat for 6–8 minutes until the sauce has thickened, then season with a pinch of salt.

Season the Savoy cabbage to taste again with salt, arrange on two plates, place the chicken legs on top, and serve with the sauce.

MARINATED PORK NECK STEAKS WITH STAR ANISE

FOR THE STEAKS

1 star anise
½ teaspoon black peppercorns
pinch of ground cinnamon
2 pinches of ground ginger
1 teaspoon medium-hot mustard
3 tablespoons olive oil
zest and juice of ½ orange
2 pork neck steaks (3½ oz/100 g each)
3 teaspoons coconut oil
salt

FOR THE VEGETABLES

4 teaspoons butter
2 yellow pepper, slices into ¾ in
    (2 cm) cubes
⅓ cup (50 g) frozen peas
salt

Serves 2
Preparation: approx. 20 minutes
Marinating: approx. 1 hour
Per portion: 525 kcal, 20 g protein,
45 g fat, 9 g carbohydrate

Crush the star anise and peppercorns together using a pestle and mortar until finely ground. Stir these in a bowl with the cinnamon, ground ginger, mustard, olive oil, ½ teaspoon of salt, and the orange zest and juice. Marinate the pork steaks in this mixture, covered in the refrigerator for at least 1 hour but ideally overnight.

Put the butter in a pan over medium heat and sauté the peppers, uncovered, for 2 minutes. Add the frozen peas and continue cooking for 3 minutes.

Meanwhile, add the coconut oil to a pan over medium heat. Take the steaks out of their marinade and let them drain slightly. Fry each one for 3 minutes on each side.

Season the vegetables to taste with salt and divide between two plates. Arrange the steaks on top and serve.

RIBEYE STEAK WITH SAUERKRAUT AND CREAMY CABBAGE

FOR THE CREAMY CABBAGE
10½ oz (300 g) sauerkraut
4 teaspoons butter
1¾ oz (50 g) celery root, peeled and
    roughly grated
scant ½ cup (100 ml) vegetable stock
¼ cup (50 g) cream
2 juniper berries, crushed or finely
    chopped
1 bay leaf
½ teaspoon dried thyme
½ teaspoon mild ground paprika
salt

FOR THE STEAKS
2 ribeye steaks (approx. 5 oz/150 g each)
3 teaspoons coconut oil
salt and pepper

Serves 2
Preparation: approx. 30 minutes
Per portion: approx. 560 kcal,
    29 g P, 47 g F, 2 g CH

Toss the sauerkraut through with a fork. Put the butter in a pan over medium heat and sweat the grated celery root for 3 minutes. Add the sauerkraut and pour in the stock and cream.

Add the juniper berries to the sauerkraut along with the bay leaf, thyme, ground paprika, and a pinch of salt, cover, and cook over low heat for 20 minutes.

Just before the sauerkraut is ready, season the steaks on both sides with salt and pepper. Add the coconut oil to a pan over high heat. Put the steaks in the pan, reduce to medium heat, and fry for 3 minutes on each side. Remove the steaks from the pan, wrap them in aluminum foil, and let rest for 5 minutes.

Meanwhile, remove the lid from the sauerkraut and let it bubble over high heat until the liquid has begun to reduce to a thicker, creamy consistency. Remove the bay leaf and serve the creamy cabbage on two plates with the steaks next to it.

BAKED LEEKS WITH MUSHROOM GRATIN

1 large leek, halved lengthwise and
    sliced into 2-in (5–6-cm) long
    sections
4 teaspoons butter, plus extra
    for greasing
3¹⁄₃ cups (300 g) button mushrooms,
    halved or quartered
scant ½ cup (100 g) cream
3½ oz (100 g) Gouda, roughly grated
½ teaspoon dried thyme
freshly grated nutmeg
sprig of thyme, roughly chopped
salt and pepper

Serves 2
Preparation: approx. 20 minutes
Cooking: approx. 30 minutes
Per portion: approx. 400 kcal,
21 g protein, 33 g fat, 5 g carbohydrate

Preheat the oven to 350°F (180°C) and grease a 10 × 8 in
(26 × 20 cm) baking dish. Place the leek pieces in the baking
dish with the cut surface facing up.

Add the butter to a pan over high heat and sauté the mushrooms
for 2 minutes.

Pour in the cream, bring to a boil, uncovered, and simmer for 1
minute over medium heat. Stir the Gouda swiftly into the cream.
Add the dried thyme, season everything with nutmeg, salt, and
pepper, and pour evenly over the leeks.

Bake the leeks in the center of the oven for 30 minutes. Arrange
the leeks on two plates, garnish with thyme, and serve.

FOR A MEATY ALTERNATIVE

Of course, you can use any kind of edible mushroom
in this dish, whatever you fancy. It is also delicious with
1–2 tablespoons of chopped ham or bacon added to the recipe,
frying it in butter along with the mushrooms. This will give the
mushroom sauce a really hearty flavor.

BRAISED PORK BELLY
WITH CELERY ROOT MASH

FOR THE PORK BELLY

1 small onion, sliced

7 oz (200 g) pork belly (boneless)

¼ teaspoon ground cinnamon

½ teaspoon ground coriander

1 teaspoon ground cumin

1 garlic clove, finely chopped or crushed

1 cup (250 ml) meat stock

salt and pepper

FOR THE CELERY ROOT MASH

9 oz (250 g) celery root, peeled and diced

4 teaspoons butter

generous ¼ cup (60 g) cream

freshly grated nutmeg

salt and pepper

Serves 2

Preparation: approx. 25 minutes

Cooking: approx. 1 hour

Per portion: approx. 465 kcal, 21 g protein, 40 g fat, 5 g carbohydrate

Preheat the oven to 350°F (180°C). Place the onion in an 8-in (20-cm) square baking dish. Using a knife, score five or six incisions in the skin of the pork belly. Lay it skin-side down on the onion and season with salt and pepper. Transfer to the center of the oven and bake for 15 minutes.

Stir the cinnamon, coriander, cumin, and garlic into the meat stock. Turn the pork belly so the skin is facing up and pour over the stock. Cook in the oven for a further 45 minutes, using a ladle to occasionally spoon some of the juices over the meat. Increase the oven temperature to 450°F (225°C) for the final 15 minutes.

Cover the celery root with water in a saucepan, season with salt and cook for 20 minutes until soft, then drain.

Heat the butter and cream in a small pan and add a pinch of nutmeg. Add the celery root, warm briefly, and process with a hand blender to make a creamy purée. Season to taste with salt and pepper.

Serve the purée on two plates. Remove the pork belly from the oven, slice crosswise into eight thin slices and arrange these alongside the celery root mash. Season the juices to taste with salt and pepper to serve.

TRY BRAISED NECK OF PORK

You could replace the pork belly with the same quantity of pork neck. Prepare the meat in the same way as the pork belly. Then add 1 tablespoon of coconut oil to a pan over medium heat. Season the pork neck with salt and pepper and fry it for 3 minutes on each side. Arrange the onions in the baking dish, lay the neck of pork on top and proceed as described in the recipe.

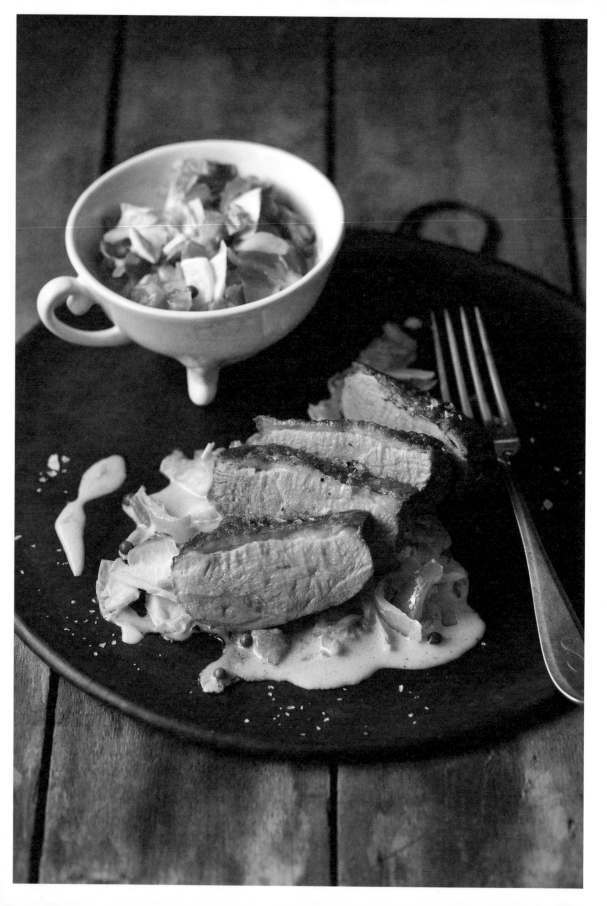

DUCK BREAST ON
A BED OF CHICORY

7 oz (200 g) Barbary duck breast
4 teaspoons clarified butter
1 small red onion, finely diced
2 tomatoes, diced
2 chicory, halved and sliced into roughly
    ½ in (1 cm) strips
scant ½ cup (100 g) cream
1 teaspoon green peppercorns in brine
salt and pepper

Serves 2
Preparation: approx. 25 minutes
Per portion: approx. 445 kcal, 21 g
protein, 36 g fat, 7 g carbohydrate

Using a sharp knife, score five or six slight incisions in the skin of the duck breast. Season the skin with salt and pepper.

Add the clarified butter to a pan over medium heat. Place the duck breast in the pan, skin-side down, and fry for 8 minutes. Season the meat side with salt and pepper, turn the duck breast over, and continue frying skin-side up for a further 6 minutes. Remove the duck breast, wrap in aluminum foil, and let rest for 8 minutes.

Meanwhile, sauté the onion in the duck fat for 1 minute. Stir in the diced tomato and the chicory, then pour in the cream. Add the green peppercorns with a bit of brine and simmer everything over high heat, stirring occasionally, until the liquid has reduced to a creamy sauce. Remove from the heat immediately, season generously with salt and pepper, and transfer to two plates.

Carve the duck breast into 10–12 slices and arrange these on the chicory to serve.

TRY WITH CHINESE CABBAGE

Although chicory has its fans, some people are not so keen on its slightly bitter flavor. If this bitter leaf is not one of your favorite vegetables, just replace it with ½ head of Chinese cabbage. You could also try replacing the green peppercorns with 1 teaspoon of capers. This gives the dish a very different, but equally delicious, flavor.

HALLOUMI WITH PAPAYA
AND TOMATO SALSA

(V)

FOR THE ZUCCHINI SALAD

1 small zucchini

1 tablespoon white wine vinegar

½ teaspoon medium-hot mustard

3 teaspoons olive oil

½ teaspoon dried thyme

salt and pepper

FOR THE SALSA

1 tomato, cubed

½ small papaya, deseeded and finely diced

1 small red onion, finely diced

1 mild red chili, deseeded and finely diced

4 basil leaves, sliced into thin strips

1 teaspoons ajvar

salt and pepper

FOR THE HALLOUMI

3 tablespoons olive oil

5 oz (150 g) halloumi

Serves 2

Preparation: approx. 30 minutes

Per portion: approx. 515 kcal,

19 g protein, 43 g fat, 7 g carbohydrate

To make the zucchini salad, first wash the zucchini, trim off the ends and grate roughly. Toss in the white wine vinegar, mustard, olive oil, and thyme. Season to taste with salt and pepper, cover, and let infuse in the refrigerator.

For the salsa, mix the tomato, papaya, red onion, chili, and basil well in the ajvar and season with salt and pepper.

Put the olive oil for the halloumi into a non-stick pan over medium heat. Cut the halloumi into two equally thick slices and fry these for 2 minutes on both sides until golden brown.

Divide the zucchini salad between two plates, arrange the halloumi on top, and serve with the papaya and tomato salsa.

ZUCCHINI AND HALLOUMI KEBABS

To make these, first slice 1 small zucchini in half lengthwise then cut it into ¾ in (2 cm) chunks. Chop 5 oz (150 g) halloumi into similar bitesize pieces and slide these alternately onto two wooden skewers with the zucchini pieces. Heat 2 tablespoons olive oil in a non-stick pan and fry each skewer for 1 minute on each side.

CAULIFLOWER RISOTTO

1 lb 5 oz (600 g) cauliflower florets
²/₃ cup (150 g) cream
4 teaspoons butter
1 small onion, finely diced
1 teaspoon curry powder
¾ cup (200 ml) vegetable stock
2 tablespoons sliced almonds
1 tablespoon almond nut butter
¾ oz (20 g) Parmesan, finely grated
3 sprigs of parsley, finely chopped
salt and pepper

Serves 2
Preparation: approx. 30 minutes
Per portion: approx. 600 kcal, 21 g
protein, 50 g fat, 16 g carbohydrate

Bring 2 cups (500 ml) water to a boil in a pan and add salt. Add a quarter of the cauliflower florets to the pan, cover, and cook for 10 minutes before draining in a sieve and transferring to a blender. Add the cream and process everything to a fine purée.

Blitz the remaining cauliflower florets in a food processor until you have crumbs resembling grains of rice. Add the butter to a shallow pan over medium heat and sauté the onion for 3 minutes. Then add the cauliflower crumbs and continue frying for 1 minute, stirring in the curry powder as you go. Pour in the vegetable stock, cover, and cook over the very lowest heat for 5 minutes.

Meanwhile, dry-toast the sliced almonds in a non-stick pan until golden and aromatic.

Add the cauliflower purée, almond nut butter and three quarters of the Parmesan to the cauliflower in the pan. Stir everything well and heat through for 2 minutes. Season to taste with salt and pepper.

Divide between two deep plates, garnished with sliced almonds, parsley, and the remaining Parmesan.

LEMON SHRIMP
ON CREAMED SPINACH

FOR THE SPINACH

4 teaspoons butter

10½ oz (300 g) frozen spinach, defrosted

scant ½ cup (100 g) cream

freshly grated nutmeg

salt

FOR THE SHRIMP

3 teaspoons coconut oil

9 oz (250 g) raw frozen jumbo shrimp
(peeled), defrosted

1 garlic clove, finely chopped or crushed

1 mild red chili, sliced into thin rings

zest and juice of 1 lemon

salt and pepper

Serves 2

Preparation: approx. 20 minutes

Defrosting: approx. 2 hours

Per portion: approx. 425 kcal, 29 g
protein, 34 g fat, 3 g carbohydrate

Heat the butter for the spinach in a pan. Squeeze all the liquid out of the spinach, roughly chop, and sauté for 2 minutes in the butter. Pour in the cream, season with a pinch of salt and nutmeg, and cook, uncovered, for 4 minutes over medium heat.

Meanwhile, add the coconut oil to a non-stick pan over high heat. Season the shrimp with salt and pepper. Fry them for 3 minutes on each side. Add the garlic and chili as they cook. Finally, deglaze the pan with the lemon juice. Adjust to taste with some grated lemon zest, salt, and pepper.

Arrange the spinach on two plates, place the shrimp on top, drizzle with the juices, and serve.

GENTLE DEFROSTING

It takes quite a while for shrimp and spinach to defrost. The best approach is to defrost them both overnight in the refrigerator, or for about 2 hours at room temperature. But if you're really in a hurry, the spinach can be defrosted with a bit of water in a pan over low heat, as per the instructions on the pack, and the shrimp can be immersed in hot water for 4–5 minutes. Once defrosted, let them drain well and proceed as described above.

SEA BREAM
ON GREEN ASPARAGUS

FOR THE ASPARAGUS
8 teaspoons butter
scant ½ cup (100 ml) vegetable stock
14 oz (400 g) green asparagus, sliced
    into 2 in (5 cm) pieces
freshly grated nutmeg
salt and pepper

FOR THE SEA BREAM
2 sea bream fillets, skin on (approx. 3½
    oz/100 g each)
1 tablespoon coconut oil
salt and pepper

FOR THE TOMATO SAUCE
2 tablespoons coconut oil
1 small onion, finely diced
1 celery stalk, finely diced
3½ oz (100 g) tomato puree
1 teaspoon mild ground paprika
salt and pepper

Serves 2
Preparation: approx. 25 minutes
Per portion: approx. 430 kcal, 24 g
protein, 34 g fat, 7 g carbohydrate

Heat the butter and vegetable stock in a shallow pan. Season with nutmeg, salt, and pepper and bring to a boil. Add the asparagus, cover, and cook over low heat for 15 minutes.

Meanwhile, season the skin side of the sea bream fillets with salt and pepper. Add the coconut oil to a pan over medium heat. Fry the sea bream fillets skin side down for 1 minute, remove from the pan, and set aside.

For the tomato sauce, add the coconut oil and diced onion to a pan and sauté for 2 minutes. Then add the celery and continue frying for 2 minutes. Pour in the puree, bring to a boil, and simmer for 3–4 minutes. Add the ground paprika and season with salt and pepper.

Place the sea bream fillets, skin side up in the sauce and cook for 2 minutes until done.

Arrange the asparagus on two plates. Place the sea bream fillets on top and serve with the tomato sauce.

BUYING SEA BREAM

Help preserve natural fish stocks by opting for farmed sea bream. Another benefit: thanks to the special food given to farmed bream, they are rich in omega-3 fatty acids with proportionately fewer omega-6 fatty acids. Omega-3 levels can be double those found in wild sea bream!

SQUID WITH PAPAYA SALSA

FOR THE SALSA

½ small papaya, peeled, deseeded and
   cubed
1 small red onion, finely diced
1 mild red chili, sliced into very thin rings
juice of ½ lemon
¼ apple, grated
4 teaspoons rapeseed oil
salt and pepper

FOR THE SQUID

4 teaspoons butter
1 garlic clove, finely chopped or crushed
10½ oz (300 g) frozen spinach, defrosted
freshly grated nutmeg
4 teaspoons coconut oil
7 oz (200 g) raw frozen squid tubes
   (ready prepared), defrosted and
   sliced into ½-in (1-cm) wide rings
salt and pepper

Serves 2
Preparation: approx. 20 minutes
Defrosting: approx. 2 hours
Per portion: approx. 415 kcal, 22 g
protein, 30 g fat, 7 g carbohydrate

Stir together the papaya, onion, chili, lemon juice, apple, and
rapeseed oil. Season to taste with salt and pepper.

Heat the butter in a pan and sweat the garlic for 1 minute.
Squeeze the spinach slightly and add to the pan. Season with a
pinch of nutmeg, salt, and pepper. Cover and cook over low heat
for 5 minutes.

Add the coconut oil to a pan over high heat. Season the squid
rings with salt and pepper and sauté them for 2–3 minutes,
stirring constantly.

Divide the spinach between two plates, arrange the squid rings
on top, and serve with the papaya salsa.

TENDER SQUID

Squid can easily become tough when cooked. The freezing
process helps make the frozen product more tender to start with.
If using fresh squid, it's best to bash them before cooking, as you
would with schnitzel. For roasting, grilling, or frying the trick is
speed and heat. For boiling, stewing, or braising I recommend
lower temperatures and similarly short cooking times to avoid
the squid developing a rubbery consistency.

REDFISH ON ZUCCHINI NOODLES

FOR THE ZUCCHINI
NOODLES
2 zucchini, spiralized (or peeled into
    tagliatelle-style strips)
3 tablespoons olive oil
1 small onion, finely sliced
salt and pepper

FOR THE REDFISH
8 teaspoons butter
2 redfish fillets (approx.
    3½ oz/100 g each)
2 tablespoons sliced almonds
½ teaspoon dried thyme
salt and pepper

Serves 2
Preparation: approx. 20 minutes
Per portion: approx. 515 kcal, 25 g
protein, 44 g fat, 5 g carbohydrate

Add the zucchini spaghetti or tagliatelle to a bowl with
½ teaspoon salt and carefully toss with your hands. Leave for 10
minutes to draw out the water, then transfer to a sieve to drain.

Put the olive oil in a pan over medium heat and sauté the
onion for 1–2 minutes until it has colored slightly. Add the
zucchini noodles and continue cooking, uncovered and stirring
occasionally, for 3–4 minutes.

Heat the butter in a non-stick pan. Season the redfish fillets with
salt and pepper. Fry the fish for 2 minutes on each side, then
remove from the pan.

Season the zucchini noodles to taste with salt and pepper and
serve on two plates. Arrange the redfish fillets on top. Add the
sliced almonds and thyme to the butter in the pan and stir.
Drizzle this over the fish to serve.

VEGETABLE NOODLES

You can create spaghetti or tagliatelle using a spiralizer or peeler
from other vegetables as well as zucchini. Long vegetables such
as cucumbers and carrots are ideal, as are round kohlrabi or
beets. Of course, you could also simply slice or dice the zucchini
and sauté them in olive oil—but dishes that are pleasing to the
eye somehow taste even better.

MONKFISH IN AN ORANGE
AND PEPPER SAUCE

FOR THE MONKFISH

3 teaspoons coconut oil

1 monkfish fillet (approx. 10½ oz/300 g),
     sliced into 6 equal pieces

1 small onion, finely diced

juice of 1 orange

scant ½ cup (100 ml) vegetable stock

1 teaspoon black peppercorns (or
     ¼ teaspoon ground black pepper)

generous ¼ cup (60 g) cream

salt and pepper

FOR THE SALAD

2 tablespoons white wine vinegar

½ teaspoon mustard

4½ tablespoons olive oil

1 handful arugula, cut into
     bitesize pieces

¼ head iceberg lettuce, thinly sliced

½ radicchio, thinly sliced

salt and pepper

Serves 2

Preparation: approx. 30 minutes

Per portion: approx. 535 kcal, 33 g
protein, 47 g fat, 8 g carbohydrate

Add the oil to a pan over medium heat, season the monkfish with salt and pepper, and sauté for 1 minute on each side. Remove and set aside on a plate.

Add the onion to the pan and sauté for 2 minutes. Pour in the orange juice and vegetable stock and bring to a boil. Roughly crush the peppercorns using a pestle and mortar, add these to the stock, and simmer, uncovered, over medium heat for 8–10 minutes.

Meanwhile, stir together the vinegar, mustard, and olive oil and season to taste with salt and pepper.

Stir the cream into the orange and pepper sauce, then reduce over high heat until the sauce begins to thicken. Remove from the heat immediately and season to taste with salt.

Toss the salad with the dressing in a bowl. Heat the monkfish medallions in the sauce for 1 minute, divide the salad between two plates, arrange the medallions on top, and serve with the sauce.

TRY WITH ARUGULA AND TOMATO SALAD

Cut 1 handful of arugula into bitesized pieces. Add 2 tablespoons of olive oil to a small pan over medium heat. Braise ⅔ cup (100 g) cherry tomatoes, halved, in the hot oil for 5 minutes, stirring occasionally. Season to taste with salt and pepper, fold into the arugula, and serve straight away with the monkfish.

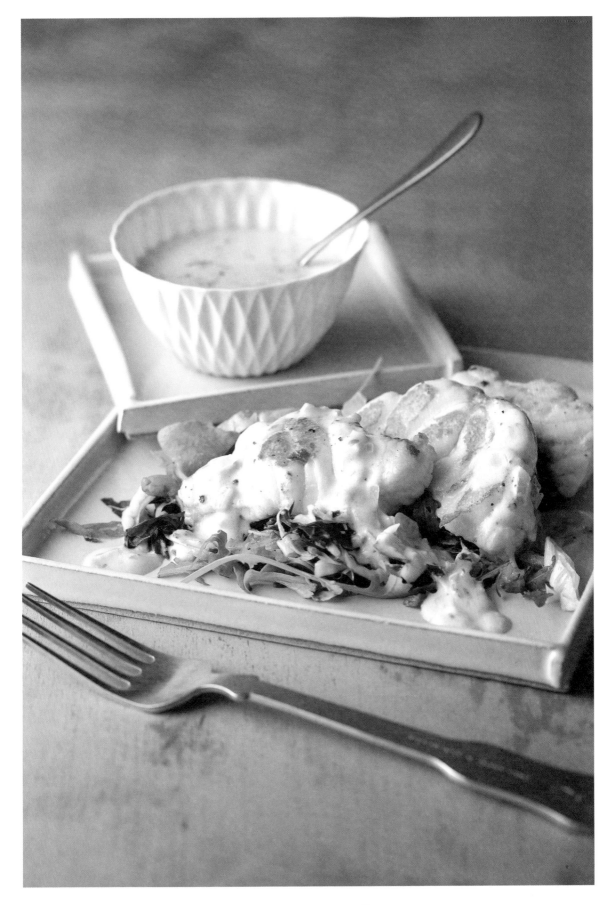

5

SNACKS

You may need a top-up, an emergency bite, or just something to keep you going. You can also use these recipes as quick and easy-to-prepare mini meals in place of larger recipes.

MINI EGGPLANT PIZZAS

1 eggplant, cut into 12 × ⅝-in (1½-cm)
   thick slices
3 tablespoons olive oil
1 teaspoon oregano
⅓ cup (80 g) chopped tomatoes (canned)
4½ oz (125 g) ball mozzarella, drained
   and sliced into 12 pieces
1½ oz (40 g) goat cheese
12 basil leaves
salt and pepper

Serves 2
Preparation: approx. 15 minutes
Cooking: approx. 30 minutes
Per portion: approx. 370 kcal, 16 g
protein, 32 g fat, 4 g carbohydrate

Preheat the oven to 400°F (200°C). Line a baking tray with
parchment paper. Brush the eggplant slices on each side with
the olive oil, lay them on the baking tray, and season on both
sides with a bit of salt. Transfer to the center of the oven and
bake for 20 minutes.

Meanwhile, add the oregano to the tomatoes and season with
salt and pepper.

Remove the baked eggplant slices from the oven and spread the
tomatoes evenly on top. Add a piece of mozzarella to each one
and crumble over the goat cheese. Continue baking for another
10 minutes.

Remove the "pizzas" from the oven and garnish each with a basil
leaf to serve.

ALTERNATIVE MINI PIZZAS

These pizzas also work brilliantly using kohlrabi or daikon radish,
which have strong, aromatic flavors. For this option, peel the
kohlrabi or radish, cut it into ¼–⅝-in (6–8 mm) thick slices
and cook for about 6 minutes in salted water. Blanch briefly in
ice-cold water, dab dry, and proceed with the rest of the
ingredients as described above.

PARMESAN AND ZUCCHINI PATTIES WITH RED PESTO

FOR THE PESTO

2 tablespoons (20 g) pine nuts

1 garlic clove, peeled

¾ oz (20 g) Parmesan, finely grated

6 basil leaves

1¾ oz (50 g) dried tomatoes (in oil),
    drained and roughly chopped

4½ tablespoons olive oil

salt and pepper

FOR THE PATTIES

1 zucchini (approx. 10½ oz/300 g),
    roughly grated

1 carrot (approx. 3½ oz/100 g), peeled
    and roughly grated

1¾ oz (50 g) Parmesan, roughly grated

1 medium egg

1 teaspoon ground psyllium husks

salt and pepper

Serves 2

Preparation: approx. 25 minutes

Cooking: approx. 20 minutes

Per portion: approx. 590 kcal, 20 g
protein, 53 g fat, 8 g carbohydrate

To make the pesto, toast the pine nuts in a dry pan over medium heat until they become fragrant. Add the garlic to a blender along with the Parmesan, basil, dried tomatoes, pine nuts, and olive oil. Blend to a fine purée. Season to taste with salt and pepper.

Preheat the oven to 400°F. Line a baking tray with parchment paper. Squeeze the liquid from the zucchini and carrot thoroughly in a clean dish towel. Swiftly mix the vegetables by hand with the Parmesan, egg, and ground psyllium husks. Season with a pinch of salt and pepper and let sit for 5 minutes.

Scoop 10 tablespoons of mixture on the baking tray, spaced slightly apart. Press each one slightly flat. Slide the tray into the center of the oven and bake the patties for 20 minutes until the edges are golden brown.

Remove from the oven and let the patties cool slightly on the tray for 5 minutes. Arrange on two plates and serve with the pesto.

PESTO FOR THE STORE CUPBOARD

Making just a small quantity of pesto is barely worth the effort. Why not stock up and quadruple the amount? The pesto will keep for several weeks if stored in a sterile jar in the refrigerator. It also tastes great with a piece of pan-fried or grilled fish.

EASY PEASY
EGG SALAD

6 medium eggs
3 tablespoons (50 g) mayonnaise
3 tablespoons (50 g) Greek yogurt
3 sprigs of parsley, finely chopped,
    some reserved for garnish
1 teaspoon curry powder
salt and pepper

Serves 2
Preparation: approx. 15 minutes
Per portion: approx. 445 kcal, 20 g
protein, 39 g fat, 3 g carbohydrate

Boil the eggs over medium heat for 8 minutes to hard-boil. Immerse in cold water and let cool.

Stir together the mayonnaise, yogurt, parsley, and curry powder until well combined.

Peel and chop the eggs. Fold the chopped egg into the mayonnaise and yogurt mixture. Season to taste with salt and pepper, garnish with the reserved parsley, and serve.

STUFFED EGGS
WITH BACON

6 medium eggs
3 strips bacon, finely diced
2½ tablespoons (40 g) mayonnaise
2 dried tomatoes (in oil), drained and
    chopped finely
2 scallions, sliced into thin rings
salt and pepper

Serves 2
Preparation: approx. 15 minutes
Per portion: approx. 455 kcal, 22 g
protein, 40 g fat, 2 g carbohydrate

Boil the eggs over medium heat for 8 minutes to hard-boil. Immerse in cold water and let cool.

Fry the bacon in a dry pan for 6 minutes until crisp.

Peel the eggs, slice in half lengthwise, and scoop out the yolk with a teaspoon. Mash the yolk with a fork and stir it together with the mayonnaise, bacon, tomatoes, and scallions. Season to taste with salt and pepper, then use a teaspoon or piping bag to fill the halved and hollowed out eggs with the mixture.

EGG CARPACCIO
WITH DIP

(V)

6 medium eggs
juice of ½ lemon
3 tablespoons (50 g) mayonnaise
2 tablespoons (30 g) cream
a bunch of chives, snipped into
    little rings
2 radishes, roughly grated
salt and pepper

Serves 2
Preparation: approx. 25 minutes
Per portion: approx. 465 kcal, 20 g
protein, 41 g fat, 3 g carbohydrate

Boil the eggs over medium heat for 8 minutes to hard-boil. Immerse in cold water and let cool.

Mix the lemon juice with the mayonnaise, cream, chives, and radishes. Season to taste with salt and pepper.

Peel the eggs and cut into ¼-in (5-mm) thick slices. Arrange the slices in a fan pattern on two plates. Drizzle with the chive dip to serve.

EGGS BAKED
IN TOMATOES

4 teaspoons coconut oil
6 tomatoes
6 basil leaves
1½ oz (40 g) Parmesan, finely grated
2 medium eggs
2½ tablespoons cream
freshly grated nutmeg
2 oz (60 g) feta, cut into 6 cubes
salt and pepper

Serves 2
Preparation: approx. 15 minutes
Cooking: approx. 25 minutes
Per portion: approx. 385 kcal,
21 g protein, 30 g fat, 6 g carbohydrate

Preheat the oven to 400°F (200°C). Grease an 8-in (20-cm) square baking dish with 1 teaspoon of the oil. Slice a lid off each tomato. Hollow them out, place in the baking dish, and insert 1 basil leaf.

Whisk the Parmesan with the eggs, cream, and remaining coconut oil. Season with salt, pepper, and nutmeg and divide between the tomatoes. Bake in the center of the oven for 8 minutes.

Place 1 cube of feta on each tomato, then continue baking for a further 13–17 minutes.

KOHLRABI FRIES WITH STRAWBERRY KETCHUP

(V)

FOR THE KOHLRABI FRIES
3 tablespoons coconut oil, melted
1 teaspoon mild ground paprika
1 teaspoon curry powder
1 large kohlrabi, cut into ⅜-in
     (8-mm) batons
salt and pepper

FOR THE KETCHUP
⅓ cup (50 g) strawberries, hulled
1 tablespoon tomato purée
1 teaspoon white wine vinegar
1 small red chili, halved and deseeded
salt and pepper

Serves 2
Preparation: approx. 20 minutes
Cooking: approx. 20 minutes
Per portion: approx. 160 kcal, 2 g protein,
15 g fat, 5 g carbohydrate

Preheat the oven to 440°F (250°C). Line a baking tray with parchment paper. Stir together the melted coconut oil, ground paprika, curry powder, 1 teaspoon of salt, and a pinch of pepper in a bowl. Add the kohlrabi batons and mix well until they are evenly coated.

Spread the kohlrabi fries over the baking tray, making sure they touch each other as little as possible. Slide the tray into the center of the oven and bake for 20 minutes. Turn the fries after 10 minutes to ensure they brown evenly.

Meanwhile, add the strawberries to a blender with the tomato purée, vinegar, and chili. Blend everything well and season to taste with salt and pepper.

Remove the kohlrabi fries from the oven and serve with the strawberry ketchup.

SUBSTITUTE WITH SQUASH
Try making these fries with a hokkaido squash, or maybe a daikon radish, instead of the kohlrabi. Both are prepared in the same way. These fries are also a fantastic side dish.

CRISPY ZUCCHINI
WITH HERB AIOLI

(V)

FOR THE AIOLI
1½ teaspoons milk
¼ cup (50 ml) olive oil
1 medium egg yolk
1 garlic clove, roughly chopped
1 tablespoon dried Italian herbs
salt and pepper

FOR THE ZUCCHINI
1 medium egg
¾ oz (20 g) Parmesan, finely grated
⅓ cup (30 g) ground almonds
1 teaspoon mild paprika
1 teaspoon dried thyme
1 large zucchini, sliced into ⅜-in
    (8-mm) thick discs
3 tablespoons coconut oil
salt

Serves 2
Preparation: approx. 20 minutes
Per portion: approx. 580 kcal, 14 g
protein, 57 g fat, 3 g carbohydrate

Peel and roughly chop the garlic. Add the milk, olive oil, and egg yolk to a blender. Slowly blend in pulses until the mixture has thickened to form a kind of mayonnaise.

Add the garlic and herbs to the mayonnaise and mix again. Season to taste with salt and pepper.

Whisk the egg in a deep bowl. Mix the Parmesan with the ground almonds, paprika, thyme, and a pinch of salt in a second bowl. First dip the zucchini slices in the egg, then coat both sides with the almond mixture.

Add the oil to a non-stick pan over medium heat. Fry the coated zucchini slices in the hot oil on each side for 2 minutes until golden brown.

Remove and let drain on paper towel before arranging on two plates. Serve with the herb aioli.

AIOLI WITHOUT EGG

If you prefer to avoid raw eggs, there is a simple alternative. If all the ingredients are puréed with a hand blender, they will thicken and combine even without the raw egg yolk. Insert the hand blender into the beaker and only switch it on when it is immersed, then slowly raise and lower it. However, the mixture will only keep its consistency for a few minutes. So, if you choose the egg-free version, it's best to make the aioli right before serving.

"QUATTRO FORMAGGI" MUFFINS

⅓ cup (50 g) almonds
⅓ cup (50 g) cashew nuts
1 oz (30 g) dried tomatoes (in oil),
    drained
a small bunch of basil, leaves picked
1¾ oz (50 g) Parmesan, finely grated
1¾ oz (50 g) Gouda, roughly grated
1¾ oz (50 g) mozzarella, roughly grated
heaping ½ cup (150 g) quark
    (40 % fat)
4 medium eggs
1 teaspoon baking powder
salt and pepper

Makes 12
Preparation: approx. 25 minutes
Baking: approx. 20 minutes
Per muffin: approx. 170 kcal, 10 g
protein, 13 g fat, 2 g carbohydrate

Preheat the oven to 350°F. Line a 12-hole muffin tin with paper cases.

Finely grind the almonds and cashew nuts in a food processor. Add the dried tomatoes and basil leaves and blitz again to a fine consistency.

Add the cheeses to a bowl along with the nut mixture and quark. Add the eggs and baking powder and combine everything well. Season with salt and pepper and divide the mixture evenly between the muffin cases.

Slide the tray into the center of the oven and bake for 20 minutes. Remove and let cool briefly. Take the muffins out of the tray and serve still warm, or leave them to cool and store in an airtight container.

CHANGE UP THE CHEESE
Why not replace the mozzarella with the same quantity of soft goat cheese or blue cheese?

BEET CHIPS WITH SOUR CREAM AND ONION

(V)

FOR THE CHIPS

1 beet

3 teaspoons olive oil

salt and pepper

FOR THE DIP

1 scallion, halved lengthwise then sliced
 into thin crescents

3 sprigs of parsley, finely chopped

scant ¼ cup (50 g) crème fraîche

1 tablespoon quark (40 % fat)

salt and pepper

Serves 2

Preparation: approx. 15 minutes

Cooking: approx. 40 minutes

Per portion: approx. 215 kcal, 3 g protein,
19 g fat, 8 g carbohydrate

Preheat the oven to 300°F (150°C) on the fan setting. Line a baking tray with parchment paper. Peel the beet (see below). Using a mandoline or slicer, create very thin rounds from the beet (⅛in/2 mm). Add these to a bowl and mix well with olive oil and a pinch of salt and pepper.

Lay the slices individually on the baking tray. Transfer to the center of the oven and bake for 20 minutes. Turn them and continue cooking for 20 minutes. During this process, open the oven door briefly every 10 minutes to allow any moisture to escape.

Meanwhile, prepare the dip. In a bowl, stir together the scallions, parsley, crème fraîche, and quark and season to taste with salt and pepper.

After 40 minutes, test whether the beet chips are sufficiently crisp. If not, reduce the oven temperature to 200°F (100°C) and let the chips dry out for another 20 minutes with the oven door slightly ajar. Serve the chips in two bowls with the dip alongside.

PREPARING BEETS

Beet juice produces stubborn stains, so you should ideally wear household gloves when peeling them. You can buy a mandoline for very little money, but if you are really skilled using a knife, you can cut wafer-thin beet slices freehand.

LEFTOVERS

Juice any leftover beets, or dress with orange and olive oil for a delicious salad.

SPINACH MUFFINS
WITH BACON

3 teaspoons coconut oil
10 strips bacon, finely chopped
1 small onion, finely diced
1 garlic clove, finely chopped or crushed
7 oz (200 g) frozen spinach, defrosted
5 medium eggs
¼ cup (30 g) coconut flour
1 teaspoon baking powder
freshly grated nutmeg
12 cherry tomatoes, halved
salt and pepper

Makes 12
Preparation: approx. 20 minutes
Baking: approx. 20 minutes
Defrosting: approx. 2 hours
Per muffin: approx. 80 kcal, 5 g protein, 6 g fat, 1 g carbohydrate

Preheat the oven to 350°F (180°C). Line a 12-hole muffin tin with paper cases.

Put the coconut oil in a pan over medium heat and fry the bacon for about 3 minutes. Add the onion and garlic and continue cooking for another 3 minutes until golden brown.

Meanwhile, squeeze the spinach, chop roughly, and mix with the eggs, coconut flour, and baking powder. Add the fried onion and bacon mixture, mix, and season with salt, pepper, and freshly grated nutmeg.

Divide the mixture evenly between the muffin cases. Put two cherry tomato halves on each muffin. Slide the tray into the center of the oven and bake the muffins for 20 minutes. Remove from the oven and let cool briefly. Take the muffins out of the tin and serve while still warm, or let cool and store in an airtight container in the refrigerator.

BREAKFAST MUFFINS WITH SALMON
For Sunday breakfast, you could replace the bacon with the same quantity of smoked salmon. Unlike the bacon, the salmon doesn't need frying. Just dice it finely and fold it into the spinach mixture at the end with the sautéed onion.

MINI BELL PEPPERS
WITH CREAM CHEESE

6 mini bell peppers
¾ oz (20 g) Parmesan, finely grated
scant ⅓ cup (80 g) full-fat cream cheese
¼ cup (20 g) ground almonds
1 teaspoon dried thyme
6 strips bacon
salt and pepper

Serves 2
Preparation: approx. 15 minutes
Cooking: approx. 10 minutes
Per portion: approx. 310 kcal, 13 g
protein, 27 g fat, 4 g carbohydrate

Preheat the oven to 400°F (200°C). Line a baking tray with parchment paper. Slice a lid off each of the peppers. If necessary, remove any white membrane or seeds.

Combine the Parmesan, cream cheese, ground almonds, and thyme to create the creamy filling. Season to taste with salt and pepper.

Transfer the cream into a piping bag fitted with a round nozzle and fill each pepper up to the rim with this mixture.

Wrap a strip of bacon lengthwise around each pepper so the opening is covered. Fix the bacon in place with a toothpick. Transfer the stuffed peppers to a baking tray and bake in the center of the oven for 10 minutes. Remove from the oven and serve.

FILLING THE PEPPERS
If you don't have a piping bag to hand, you can also use a teaspoon to scoop the cream into the peppers, or you can adapt a freezer bag for this purpose by snipping off a little bit of one corner.

6

SWEET TREATS

We are not fans of sugar, but you can
find sweetness in other places. Dark chocolate
is delicious on its own, but with minimum
70% cocoa solids. Birch sugars are also good
substitutes, but not so much that you are
tempted into too many calories and offset the
keto effect.

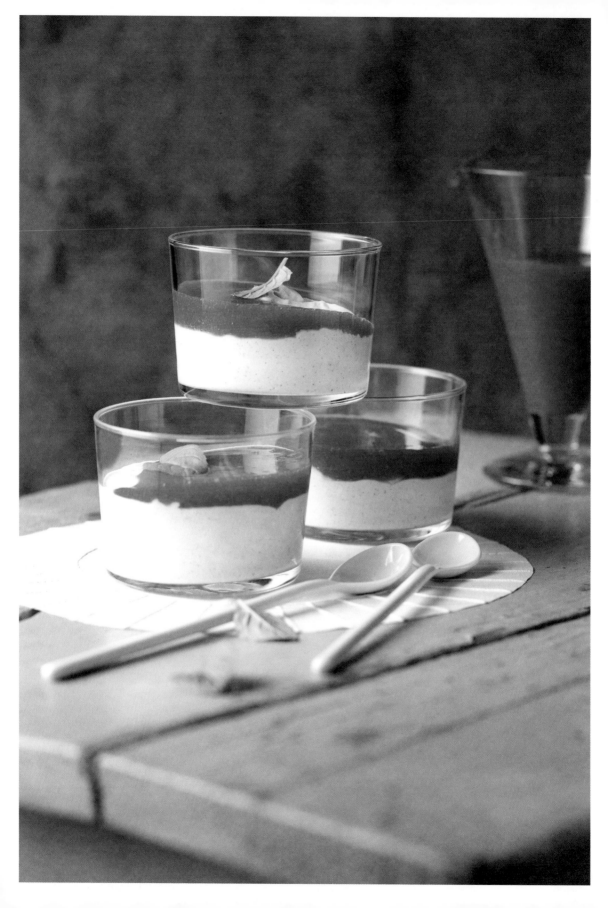

YOGURT PANNA COTTA
WITH STRAWBERRY SAUCE

FOR THE PANNA COTTA
4 sheets leaf gelatin
1 vanilla pod
²/₃ cup (150 g) cream
¼ teaspoon ground cinnamon
¾ cup (200 g) Greek yogurt
birch sugar (xylitol), optional

FOR THE STRAWBERRY SAUCE
zest and juice of ½ lime
1 cup (150 g) strawberries, hulled
4 mint leaves, to serve

Serves 2
Preparation: approx. 25 minutes
Chilling: approx. 4 hours
Per portion: approx. 390 kcal, 10 g
protein, 33 g fat, 11 g carbohydrate

Soak the gelatin for 5 minutes in ice-cold water. Meanwhile, slice the vanilla pod lengthwise and scrape out the seeds. Add both seeds and pod to a pan with the cream, cinnamon, ¼ cup (50 ml) water and bring to the boil.

Remove the gelatin from the water and squeeze it out. Stir the gelatin into the hot cream until it has completely dissolved. Remove the vanilla pod, stir in the yogurt, and add birch sugar to taste, if desired. Divide the panna cotta between two glasses or dessert dishes. Cover and chill for at least 4 hours or overnight.

Add the lime zest and juice and strawberries to a blender and blend until smooth. Spread the strawberry purée over the panna cotta and garnish with mint leaves to serve.

TRY WITH CHOCOLATE SAUCE

To make a chocolate sauce instead of the strawberry option, finely chop or grate 1½ oz (40 g) dark chocolate (minimum 70% cocoa content). Bring a scant ½ cup (100 g) cream to the boil in a pan, then remove from the heat. Add the chocolate and stir until it has completely melted. Add ½ teaspoon vanilla powder and birch sugar to taste. Let the chocolate sauce cool completely before serving.

NOTE

Leaf gelatin can be purchased online.

LEMON CREAM CHEESE MUFFINS

FOR THE BASE
3¼ oz (90 g) butter
1¼ cups (120 g) almond flour
salt

FOR THE FILLING
3 medium eggs
1¼ cups (300 g) full-fat cream cheese
2 teaspoons baking powder
½ teaspoon vanilla powder
zest of 1½ lemons, ½ very thinly sliced
    to decorate
zest of ½ orange
birch sugar (xylitol), optional
salt
½ lemon, very finely sliced, to decorate

Makes 12
Preparation: approx. 20 minutes
Baking: approx. 30 minutes
Per muffin: approx. 170 kcal, 7 g protein,
15 g fat, 1 g carbohydrate

Preheat the oven to 340°F. Line a 12-hole muffin tin with paper cases.

Melt the butter and work it into the almond flour with a pinch of salt to create a crumbly consistency. Divide this crumbly mixture evenly between the muffin cases and press down firmly, so the base of each case is covered. Transfer to the center of the oven and bake for 10 minutes.

Meanwhile, stir together the eggs, cream cheese, baking powder, vanilla powder, a pinch of salt, plus the lemon and orange zest until well combined. Add some birch sugar, if desired.

Pour the mixture onto the pre-baked muffin bases and continue baking in the center of the oven for 20 minutes. Remove the muffins from the oven, let cool briefly, then remove from the tin to cool completely on a wire rack.

Decorate the muffins with the thin lemon slices.

FREEZING THE MUFFINS
These muffins freeze really well if individually protected with plastic wrap. This way you'll always have some supplies. Just defrost the frozen muffins for 10–12 minutes in an oven preheated to 400°F (200°C), or warm up defrosted muffins in the microwave or toaster, and enjoy!

LEMON AND YOGURT GELÉES

8 sheets leaf gelatin
zest and juice of 1 lemon
scant ½ cup (100 ml) apple juice
7 teaspoons olive oil
½ packet sugar-free powdered lemon
    gelatin
⅓ cup (100 g) Greek yogurt
birch sugar (xylitol), optional

Makes 20
Preparation: approx. 15 minutes
Chilling: approx. 6 hours
Per gelée: approx. 30 kcal, 1 g protein, 2
g fat, 1 g carbohydrate

Soak the leaf gelatin for 5 minutes in ice-cold water. Mix the lemon juice, apple juice, olive oil, and 1 tablespoon of water in a saucepan.

Stir in the powdered gelatin and bring to the boil, stirring occasionally, then immediately remove from the heat.

Squeeze out the leaf gelatin by hand and dissolve it in the hot liquid. Stir in the yogurt and lemon zest, and some birch sugar to taste, if desired. Divide the mixture evenly into a 20-hole silicone bundt tray. Alternatively, if you don't have a silicone mini bundt mold tray, pour the mixture into a rimmed baking sheet or baking dish.

Chill for at least 6 hours in the refrigerator until set, ideally over-night. Press out of the silicone molds or cut into servings from the baking sheet or use your favorite small cookie cutter. Store in an airtight container in the refrigerator until ready to eat. The yogurt gelées will keep, chilled, for 1 week.

RASPBERRY YOGURT GELÉES
Replace the lemon with generous ¾ cup (100 g) raspberries. Blend the raspberries with ¼ cup (50 ml) apple juice and ¼ cup (50 ml) water, then press them through a sieve to remove the seeds. Stir in ½ packet unsweetened raspberry jello and continue as described.

NOTE
Leaf gelatin can be purchased online.

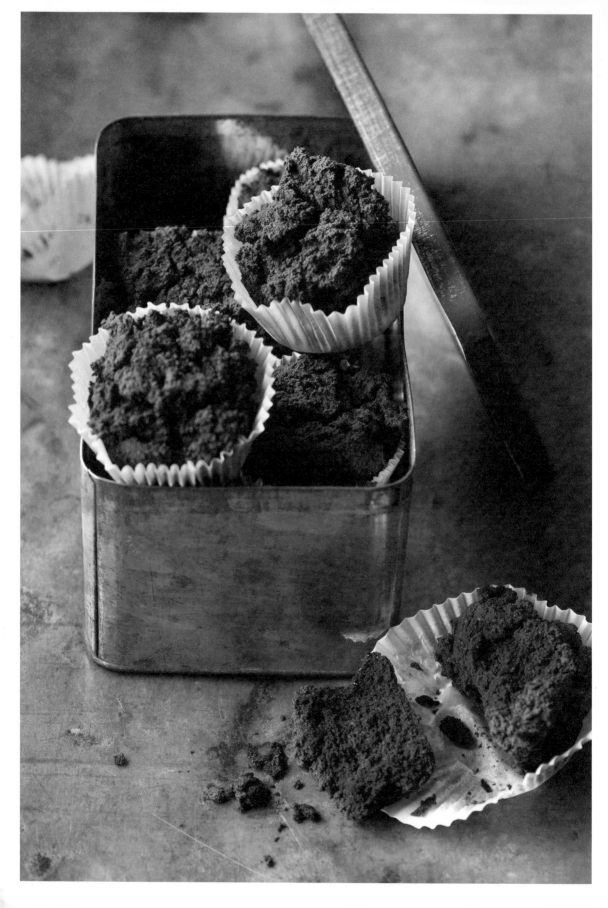

AVOCADO AND CHOCOLATE MUFFINS

scant 2 cups (180 g) almond flour
heaping ½ cup (70 g) cocoa powder
½ teaspoon baking soda
½ teaspoon baking powder
1 avocado, peeled and pitted
4 tablespoons coconut oil, melted
1 cup (280 g) Greek yogurt
2 medium eggs
½ teaspoon vanilla powder
birch sugar (xylitol), optional

Makes 12
Preparation: approx. 20 minutes
Baking: approx. 25 minutes
Per muffin: approx. 180 kcal, 9 g protein,
15 g fat, 2 g carbohydrate

Preheat the oven to 350°F (180°C). Line a 12-hole muffin tin with paper cases. Combine the almond flour, cocoa powder, baking soda, and baking powder and sift into a bowl through a sieve. Scoop the avocado flesh into a blender with the melted coconut oil, yogurt, eggs, and vanilla powder and blend until smooth. Sift the dry ingredients into the avocado mixture.

Stir until everything is well combined. Optionally, add some birch sugar to sweeten, then use a tablespoon to divide the mixture evenly between the muffin cases.

Slide the tray into the center of the oven and bake for 25 minutes. Remove, let cool briefly, then remove the muffins from the tin to cool completely on a wire rack.

TRY WITH DARK CHOCOLATE
Try the recipe with 2 oz (60 g) dark chocolate instead of the cocoa powder; this makes the muffins even more moist. For this version you will need to grate the chocolate as finely as possible. Just fold the chocolate into the mixture right at the end.

CHOCO-NUT BITES

3 oz (80 g) dark chocolate (minimum 70%
    cocoa content), finely chopped
½ cup (50 g) pecans, roughly chopped
¼ cup (30 g) almonds, roughly chopped
3½ teaspoons (10 g) hulled
    pumpkin seeds
fleur de sel (or sea salt)

Makes 6
Preparation: approx. 15 minutes
Chilling: approx. 1 hours
Per bite: approx. 165 kcal, 3 g protein, 15
g fat, 5 g carbohydrate

Line a baking tray with parchment paper. Melt the chocolate in
a little bowl suspended over a bain-marie, stirring occasionally.
Add the nuts to the melted chocolate and stir until well-coated.

Scoop six tablespoons of the chocolate and nut mixture to create
little heaps, placed slightly apart on the baking tray. Scatter the
nutty heaps with pumpkin seeds and sprinkle over a few grains
of fleur de sel.

Transfer the choco-nut bites to the refrigerator for 1 hour until
the chocolate has set. They will keep for up to 2 weeks in an
airtight container stored in the refrigerator.

CHOCOLATE COCONUT BALLS

(V)

1 avocado, peeled and pitted
heaping ⅓ cup (100 g) full-fat
   cream cheese
1¾ oz (50 g) soft butter
½ cup (60 g) coconut flour
¼ cup (30 g) cocoa powder
½ teaspoon vanilla powder
birch sugar (xylitol), optional
heaping ½ cup (60 g) ground almonds
¼ cup (20 g) desiccated coconut

Makes 20 balls
Preparation: approx. 20 minutes
Per ball: approx. 90 kcal, 2 g protein,
9 g fat, 1 g carbohydrate

Scoop the avocado flesh into a food processor. Add the cream cheese, butter, coconut flour, cocoa powder, and vanilla powder and process everything until well combined. Add some birch sugar, if desired.

Transfer to a bowl, knead in the ground almonds and let rest for 10 minutes. Shape 20 equal-size balls from the mixture using your hands and toss them in desiccated coconut. The chocolate coconut balls will keep for up to 1 week if stored in an airtight container in the refrigerator.

A DIFFERENT COATING

Instead of the desiccated coconut, try a handful of roasted, unsalted pistachios—they can be chopped up in no time and ground in a food processor and will be considerably cheaper than raw, ready-shelled pistachio kernels. Another great option for a deliciously different flavor is to use sliced almonds, chopped slightly smaller using a knife.

PEANUT BARS

7 oz (200 g) dark chocolate (minimum
     70% cocoa content), finely chopped
4 tablespoons peanut butter
     (unsweetened)
1 tablespoon butter
¾ cup (120 g) salted peanuts,
     roughly chopped
birch sugar (xylitol), optional

Makes 8 bars
Preparation: approx. 15 minutes
Chilling: approx. 4 hours
Per bar: approx. 295 kcal, 9 g protein,
24 g fat, 10 g carbohydrate

Line an 8 × 6 in (20 × 16 cm) dish with parchment
paper. Melt the chocolate in a little bowl over a bain-marie
stirring occasionally.

Combine the peanut butter with the chocolate, then stir in the
butter until it has completely melted. Finally, fold in the peanuts
until well mixed. Add some birch sugar, if desired.

Spoon into the dish, smooth the surface and chill in the
refrigerator for at least 4 hours, ideally overnight.

Use the parchment paper to lift the solid chocolate block out of
the dish, transfer to a chopping board, and slice into eight bars,
measuring roughly 3 × 1 in (8 × 3 cm). The bars will keep, chilled
in an airtight container, for up to 4 weeks.

BETTER WITHOUT SWEETENERS

If sweetened, these bars are so tempting—you can easily polish
off too many and slip out of ketosis. So it's best to not add any
sweeteners, or only make a batch when you are certain you'll be
able to resist them.

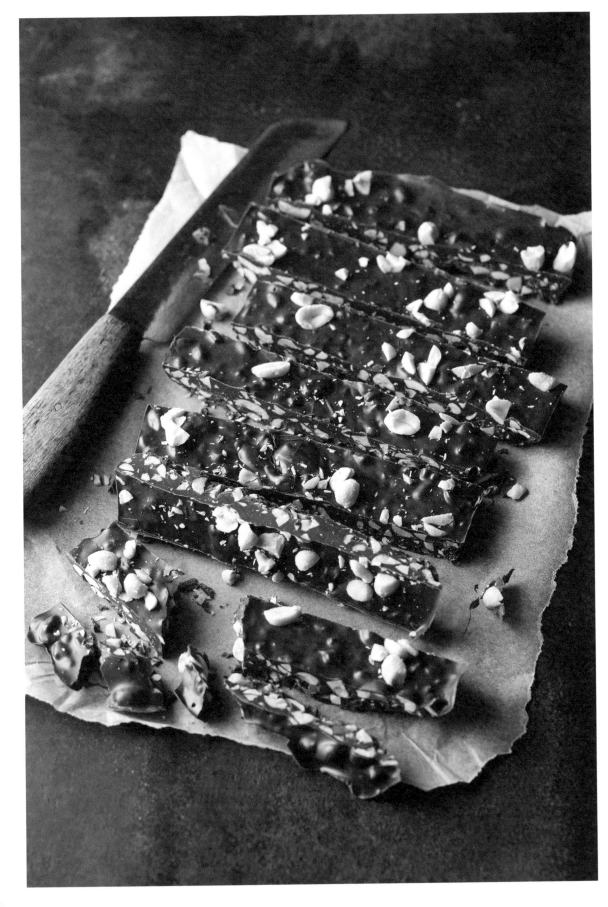

ALMOND AND
COCONUT COOKIES

2½ oz (75 g) butter
1²/₃ cups (150 g) desiccated coconut
½ cup (50 g) ground almonds
2 medium egg yolk
1 medium egg
birch sugar (xylitol), optional

Makes 15 cookies
Preparation: approx. 20 minutes
Baking: approx. 10 minutes
Per cookie: approx. 115 kcal, 1 g protein,
12 g fat, 1 g carbohydrate

Preheat the oven to 400°F. Line a baking tray with parchment paper. Melt the butter in a small pan. Combine the desiccated coconut and ground almonds with the egg yolks and egg in a bowl. Add the melted, slightly cooled butter and work everything together by hand. Add some birch sugar, if desired.

Scoop teaspoons of the cookie mix and roll into balls between the palms of your hands. Place them on the baking tray and flatten by hand until ⅜-in (8 mm) thick. Slide the tray into the center of the oven and bake for 10 minutes until the cookies are brown at the edges. Remove and let cool completely on the tray.

NUTTY COCONUT COOKIES

If you've just run out of almonds, or you have leftovers of some other nuts from another recipe, these cookies are the ideal way to use them up. Any kind of nut you happen to have in the cupboard or that needs using up can be used instead of the almonds, just grind the whole nuts in a food processor.

AVOCADO AND CHOCOLATE
ICE CREAM

(V)

1 banana, roughly chopped

1 avocado, peeled, pitted, and roughly
    chopped

scant ¼ cup (50 g) crème fraîche

2 tablespoons cocoa powder

½ teaspoon vanilla powder

1 tablespoon creamed coconut

1 tablespoon cold coffee

birch sugar (xylitol), optional

Serves 2

Preparation: approx. 10 minutes

Freezing: approx. 40 minutes

Per portion: approx. 530 kcal, 8 g protein,
49 g fat, 14 g carbohydrate

Add the banana, avocado, and crème fraîche to the bowl of
a food processor with the blade fitted. Freeze in this container
for 40–50 minutes.

Remove the food processor bowl from the freezer. Add the
cocoa powder, vanilla powder, creamed coconut, and cold coffee
and process well. Add some birch sugar to taste, if using. Serve
straight away in two little bowls.

NO ICE-CREAM MAKER REQUIRED

Normally ice cream is made by stirring it constantly in an
ice-cream maker while it is being chilled. That isn't possible
when making this ice cream. To make sure the ingredients don't
get warm too quickly when you blend them, it really helps if
the food processor bowl and blade have been frozen too. It's
worth making a bit of extra room to do this in your freezer
compartment. But be careful, ice cream can be addictive.

BULLETPROOF COFFEE

5 tablespoons ground coffee
8 teaspoons butter
3 tablespoons coconut oil

Serves 2
Preparation: approx. 10 minutes
Per serving: approx. 325 kcal, 7 g protein,
32 g fat, 1 g carbohydrate

Prepare two cups of coffee using 1¾ cup (400 ml) water and
the ground coffee. Melt the butter and coconut oil in a pan over
medium heat and warm them slightly.

Add the coffee, butter and coconut oil to a blender and process
until all the ingredients are combined and there is a nice layer
of foam. Pour into two pre-warmed cups to serve.

FOR MORE INDULGENCE

You can jazz up this coffee with some vanilla powder, ground
cinnamon, or cardamom. If you have a sweet tooth, you can use
a sweetener of your choice or just dissolve a little piece of dark
chocolate (minimum 70 % cocoa content) in your coffee. If you
like cream with your coffee, warm it up together with the butter
and coconut oil.

BULLETPROOF HOT CHOCOLATE

(V)

generous ¾ cup (200 g) coconut
    milk (canned)
5½ teaspoons soft butter
3 teaspoons coconut oil
4 tablespoons cocoa powder
¼ teaspoons vanilla powder
pinch of ground cinnamon

Serves 2
Preparation: approx. 10 minutes
Per serving: approx. 510 kcal, 12 g
protein, 49 g fat, 6 g carbohydrate

Add the coconut milk to a small pan with ¾ cup (200 ml) water
and bring to the boil. Stir in the butter, coconut oil, cocoa powder, vanilla, and cinnamon and remove the pan from the heat.

Pour the hot chocolate into a blender and process until all the ingredients have combined and there is a nice layer of foam. Pour
into two pre-warmed cups to serve.

GENERAL INDEX

RECIPE INDEX

STERLING EPICURE
New York

An Imprint of Sterling Publishing Co., Inc.
1166 Avenue of the Americas
New York, NY 10036

ISBN 978-1-4549-3602-2

Distributed in Canada by Sterling Publishing Co., Inc.
c/o Canadian Manda Group, 664 Annette Street
Toronto, Ontario, Canada M6S 2C8

For information about custom editions, special sales, and premium and corporate
purchases, please contact Sterling Special Sales at 800-805-5489 or
specialsales@sterlingpublishing.com.

Manufactured in China

2 4 6 8 10 9 7 5 3 1

sterlingpublishing.com

Photography by Mona Binner, except p.22 (Shutterstock)
Translated by Alison Tunley

Originally published under the title: *Low Carb, High Fat*
© 2017 by Gräfe und Unzer Verlag

ABOUT THE AUTHORS
Prof. Jürgen Vormann studied nutritional science at the University of Hohenheim Stuttgart) and is the founder of the
Institute for Prevention and Nutrition (Institut für Prävention und Ernährung—IPEV) near Munich. Prof. Vormann shares
his extensive knowledge about vitamins, minerals, and the acid-base balance in the introduction to this book, as well as
through lectures and television appearances.

Nico Stanitzok is a chef with a dietary background, a well-known food
blogger, and successful author of several cookbooks.